How to Keep from
Breaking Your Heart

What Every Woman Needs to Know About
Cardiovascular Disease

SECOND EDITION

Barbara H. Roberts, MD, FACC
Foreword by Meredith Vieira

JONES AND BARTLETT PUBLISHERS
Sudbury, Massachusetts
BOSTON   TORONTO   LONDON   SINGAPORE

World Headquarters

Jones and Bartlett Publishers
40 Tall Pine Drive
Sudbury, MA 01776
978-443-5000
info@jbpub.com
www.jbpub.com

Jones and Bartlett Publishers
Canada
6339 Ormindale Way
Mississauga, Ontario L5V 1J2
Canada

Jones and Bartlett Publishers
International
Barb House, Barb Mews
London W6 7PA
United Kingdom

Substantial discounts on bulk quantities of Jones and Bartlett's publications are available to corporations, professional associations, and other qualified organizations. For details and specific discount information, contact the special sales department at Jones and Bartlett via the above contact information or send an email to specialsales@jbpub.com.

Jones and Bartlett's books and products are available through most bookstores and online booksellers. To contact Jones and Bartlett Publishers directly, call 800-832-0034, fax 978-443-8000, or visit our website www.jbpub.com.

The authors, editor, and publisher have made every effort to provide accurate information. However, they are not responsible for errors, omissions, or for any outcomes related to the use of the contents of this book and take no responsibility for the use of the products and procedures described. Treatments and side effects described in this book may not be applicable to all people; likewise, some people may require a dose or experience a side effect that is not described herein. Drugs and medical devices are discussed that may have limited availability controlled by the Food and Drugs Administration (FDA) for use only in a research study or clinical trial. Research, clinical practice, and government regulations often change the accepted standard in this field. When consideration is being given to use of any drug in the clinical setting, the health care provider or reader is responsible for determining FDA status of the drug, reading the package insert, and reviewing prescribing information for the most up-to-date recommendations on dose, precautions, and contraindications, and determining the appropriate usage for the product. This is especially important in the case of drugs that are new or seldom used.

Production Credits
Publisher: Christopher Davis
Associate Editor: Kathy Richardson
Acquisitions Editor: Janice Hackenberg
Editorial Assistant: Jessica Acox
Production Director: Amy Rose
Production Editor: Daniel Stone
Associate Marketing Manager: Ilana Goddess
V.P. of Manufacturing and Inventory Control: Therese Connell
Composition: Spoke & Wheel/Jason Miranda
Cover Design: Kristin E. Ohlin
Cover Image: © Iaroslav Neliubov/ShutterStock, Inc.
Printing and Binding: Malloy, Inc.
Cover Printing: Malloy, Inc.

Library of Congress Cataloging-in-Publication Data
Roberts, Barbara.
  How to keep from breaking your heart / Barbara Roberts.
    p. cm.
  Includes bibliographical references and index.
  ISBN-13: 978-0-7637-6050-2
  ISBN-10: 0-7637-6050-1
  1. Heart diseases in women—Popular works. 2. Heart diseases in women—Miscellanea. I. Title.
  RC682.R555 2009
  616.1'20082—dc22
                              2008028610
6048

Printed in the United States of America
12 11 10 09 08   10 9 8 7 6 5 4 3 2 1

Contents

Acknowledgments

At Jones and Bartlett my appreciation goes to Janice Hackenberg and Chris Davis.

Dr. Kathleen Hittner, President and CEO of the Miriam Hospital, conceived of a center that would be devoted to the diagnosis, treatment, and prevention of cardiovascular disease in women. She and Sandra Coletta brought the center to fruition and asked me to be its medical director. I owe them both an enormous debt of gratitude. The Women's Cardiac Center staff has expanded in the years since the first edition of this book was published. Patty Shea Leary, RNP and Clinic Secretary Becky Aucoin remain, and remain the backbone of the center. They are joined by Joan Brennan, RNP, secretary Melissa Monteiro, and part-time jack-of-all trades Zara Vartanian-Hajinian, all dedicated to our mission. I would like to thank Dr. Michael Atalay for his invaluable assistance in the sections on CT angiography and Cardiac Magnetic Resonance Imaging.

My gratitude goes to my colleagues in the Division of Cardiology at the Miriam Hospital, who free up my time and energy for writing by taking night and weekend call. I am grateful to Drs. Robert Indeglia, Ken Korr, Paul Gordon, B. Greg Brown, Marianne Legato, and Paul Thompson for their friendship and guidance. Dr. Bernard Lown is an inspiring mentor and outstanding role model; no words of mine can express his importance to my development as a physician. I revere the memories of my late teachers Drs. Richard Gorlin, Robert Levy, Walter Pritchard and Austin Weisberger. Any skills I have as a healer I owe to their wise tutelage.

I can never repay the debt I owe to my parents, Dorothy and Alan Hudson, who instilled in me a love of learning and gifted me with nine younger siblings. My sisters and brothers were my first "patients" during endless games of "doctor" as a child. They and their families enrich my life in ways too numerous to write. My children, Dorie, Archie, and Meagan Roberts, are my pride and joy. My husband, Joe Avarista, is my champion in all things, my right hand, and my heart.

Last, but far from least I want to thank my patients, who humble me with their trust, inspire me with their courage, and cheer me with their affection.

Foreword

by Meredith Vieira

Why would Barbara want me to write the foreword to her book? I know next to nothing about women and heart disease. In fact I'm painfully, and dangerously, ignorant when it comes to the topic. Maybe that's why.

After all, I'm a well-educated woman who visits the homes of millions of other women every day as co-host of NBC's *The Today Show.* I pride myself on being well informed and sharing that knowledge with others. So why don't I understand my own body? Why have I, why have all of us for that matter, been kept in the dark?

No, I don't believe it's the result of some vast male conspiracy (although I've never forgiven them for creating the brassiere). But I do know that, until recently, the medical profession has ignored the physiological differences between guys and dolls when it comes to matters of the heart. Finally, doctors are beginning to get an accurate picture of women and heart disease. And it's not pretty.

I'm not trying to scare you. Or maybe I am. There's no comfort in the fact that cardiovascular disease kills more women than men. And I'm sure not thrilled to discover that being menopausal puts me at even greater risk of heart attack. But what do they say about the enemy you know? At least now, thanks in large part to people like Barbara, we can take back control of our bodies. I don't know about you, but I refuse to stay in the dark any longer.

Recently my daughter, Lily, was chosen to play the Tin Man in a local production of *The Wizard of Oz*. As I finish writing this foreword, I'm reminded of his words, and how poignant they now sound coming out of a little girl's mouth. All the Tin Man ever wanted was a heart that he could "lock with a zipper." He finally gets his wish, and as Dorothy is leaving Oz, he utters his last words to her, "Now I know I've got a heart, because it's breaking." I can't protect Lily from that kind of heartache, not with all the zippers in the world. But I can keep her from breaking her heart by teaching her what really ticks inside of her, inside of all of us.

On behalf of my "Tin Woman," I urge you to read on.

Meredith Vieira

Preface

In March 2001, at about the same time I began work on the first edition of this book, a group of some seventy experts met at the National Heart Lung and Blood Institute (NHLBI) of the National Institutes of Health (NIH). Their purpose was to develop a nationwide plan to reduce the toll that heart disease took on American women. Based on their recommendations, the NHLBI began *The Heart Truth* campaign to educate women to the fact that cardiovascular disease was their number one killer. In 2002, the Red Dress Project was launched as a centerpiece of the campaign.

The Red Dress was chosen as the symbol of the Heart Truth Campaign because, as an icon, it was cited by women for its ability to "convey the seriousness of heart disease, and change the perception that it is only a man's issue." Since 2003, each year well-known designers including Calvin Klein, Heidi Klum, Caroline Herrara, Donna Karan, and others have provided red dresses for the Red Dress Collection Fashion Show held in New York City during February, Heart Health month. The Red Dress Project quickly became a highly visible and successful public health campaign. In 2000, only one in three American women knew that heart disease was their number one killer. As a result of the widespread educational efforts spearheaded by the Heart Truth campaign and the Red Dress Project, that total had risen to 57% by 2006. Particularly during February in the last few years, it has been hard to turn on the television and not see some feature about heart disease in women.

In addition, many women's magazines have had recurring features on heart health in their pages. In February 2004, *Good Housekeeping* magazine listed 44 of the top cardiac centers for women (including ours here in Rhode Island). In March 2005, *Woman's Day* magazine profiled three centers, ours and two others in California and Missouri. The article described how "three women's heart centers help twelve women get heart smart makeovers." In addition, *Woman's Day*, under the leadership of editor-in-chief Jane Chesnutt, provides regular updates on heart disease treatment and prevention in women, with assistance from a Women's Heart Health Advisory Board on which I serve. Nor are features about women and heart disease confined to the pages of women's magazines. *Time Magazine* did a cover article on the subject in April 2003, and *Newsweek* has published many articles on women and heart disease.

While large numbers of women (and physicians) have been educated about the scope of the problem, much remains to be done. In fact, a 2005 article published in *Circulation*, the journal of the American Heart Association, pointed out how persistent are the misconceptions about cardiovascular disease, even among medical doctors. Dr. Lori Mosca and her colleagues administered online questionnaires to 500 physicians in three specialties: 100 cardiologists, 100 obstetrician-gynecologists, and 300 primary care physicians. A striking finding in this study was that only 8% of primary care physicians, 13% of obstetrician–gynecologists, and 17% of cardiologists knew that more women than men die every year from cardiovascular disease in the United States.

More research into heart disease in women has been undertaken in the years since the first edition of this book was published. New and exciting advances in our ability to prevent and treat heart disease are occurring on a regular basis. The *Second Edition* of *How To Keep From Breaking Your Heart* incorporates this new knowledge in terms accessible to the lay reader.

In February 2004, one month after the publication of the first edition of *How To Keep From Breaking Your Heart*, I received an invitation to the White House. First Lady Laura Bush invited directors of women's cardiac centers, and other people interested in heart disease in women, to a press conference and luncheon to kick off Heart Health month and publicize the Red Dress Project and The Heart Truth Campaign. At that luncheon I was able to present the First Lady with a copy of *How To Keep From Breaking Your Heart*.

Perhaps in February 2009 I will be able to hand this *Second Edition* to the new First Lady. But whether or not that occurs, it is my hope that you will find this book helpful in protecting and preserving the most important muscle in your body, your heart.

Barbara H. Roberts, MD, FACC

Introduction

A few years ago, the telephone rang in my office on a particularly busy afternoon. The caller was a doctor at a nearby hospital who wished to refer a patient to me. The patient, a 58-year-old woman, had been admitted with congestive heart failure, and the doctors taking care of her recommended that she undergo a diagnostic test called a cardiac catheterization. She told them that she would not have a heart catheterization until she could consult with me because I had been taking care of her father for a number of years, and she wanted to be sure that I agreed that this test was indicated.

When I saw her in the office a few days later, the story she told me upset me so much that I began to obsess about it. She reported that she had not seen a doctor since the birth of her last child almost thirty years ago, until three years earlier, when she noticed that her vision was becoming blurred. She saw an optometrist who referred her to an ophthalmologist, a physician who specializes in eye diseases. The ophthalmologist looked in the back of her eye and said: "You have diabetes," and referred her to an internist. Within three years, she had gone completely blind from diabetic eye disease, her kidneys had failed, requiring her to have dialysis three times every week, and she had had two silent heart attacks that left her in heart failure. I knew that every one of these complications could have been prevented, or their onset delayed, had her diabetes been diagnosed and treated promptly. Blindness and kidney failure can occur after about a decade of uncontrolled diabetes. So I was distraught because I realized that her suffering was preventable.

I knew that there were no insurance issues that might have kept my patient from seeing a physician for all those years. Her husband belonged to a very powerful union. The only people who have better health insurance than they do are the members of the United States Congress. So I began to think that my patient must have had a terrible experience with a doctor at some point in her life to have avoided the medical profession for so long.

When I could no longer stand not knowing I finally asked her: "Jane (not her real name), did you have a really bad experience with a doctor at some point? Is that why you didn't see one for so long?"

"No," she replied. "I felt fine, so I didn't think anything could be wrong with me."

I realized then and there that I needed to write this book. The sad fact is that most people feel the way my patient did: As long as they don't have symptoms, they don't have to worry. But atherosclerosis, a form of hardening of the arteries that causes most cardiovascular disease, begins in childhood and causes no symptoms until late in its course. Diabetes, which is becoming epidemic in the developed world, is a major risk factor for atherosclerosis. You can have diabetes and not know it until it is too late. You can have sky-high cholesterol, and frighteningly high blood pressure, with absolutely no symptoms. But all of these "risk factors" can result in cardiovascular disease, the number one killer of women AND men. They are all treatable, but first they must be diagnosed.

Compounding the problem for women is that they often think heart disease is not something for which they are at risk, that it is a "man's problem." They don't realize (and sadly sometimes their doctors don't either) that women may have unusual symptoms when they develop cardiovascular disease. I hadn't been in practice very long before I began to see increasing numbers of female patients who had been misdiagnosed. These women had gone from doctor to doctor with complaints that were labeled "anxiety" when in fact they were suffering from cardiovascular disease.

Why was this happening? The short answer is that their physicians were not listening to them as carefully as they should. But the true answers to this question are complex and run the gamut from ignorance to gender bias. Often the women were as much in the dark as their doctors in this regard. Both lacked the knowledge about the differences between men and women in various disease states, which is only now emerging. Both subscribed to the mistaken belief that cardiovascular disease predominantly affected men. In fact, more women than men have died of cardiovascular disease in the United States every year since 1984.

To get back to my patient, her cardiac catheterization showed such extensive blockages in the heart arteries, and such poor heart function, that she was not a candidate for bypass surgery or angioplasty (the "balloon" procedure that can open up blocked arteries). While on a trip to visit family over the Christmas holidays she suffered a stroke, followed by another heart attack, and she died. She went from first symptom to death in only three years. I will never forget her. I hope that reading this book will prevent other similar tragedies.

The *Second Edition* of *How to Keep from Breaking Your Heart: What Every Woman Needs to Know About Cardiovascular Disease* will teach you how to keep your heart healthy. Part One focuses on prevention. I discuss what cardiac risk factors are and what you can do if you have them. (It really is true that an ounce of prevention is worth a pound of cure.) In Part Two, I discuss specific heart diseases and the tests used to diagnose them. If you have been diagnosed with heart disease, Part Two will inform you about all the exciting new treatments that can prolong your life and allow you to live life to the fullest. Part Three contains interesting facts about the past and future of medicine and advice on finding a doctor you can trust.

This book distills knowledge I have gained over more than thirty years as a cardiologist. Aimed at women (and the men who love them), it will arm you with information about every weapon medicine has at its disposal to fight the nation's number one killer.

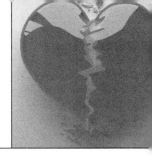

Chapter 1

The Normal Heart

The mammalian heart is the most wondrous pump that nature has devised. Even though they didn't know about its role in circulating the blood, the ancient Egyptians recognized the importance of the heart. They regarded it as the principal vital organ; it was the only organ left in position during the embalming process.

In order to keep your heart healthy, you need to know some facts about its anatomy and function. The heart starts to form in the early weeks of fetal development. It forms from a tube which folds upon itself to ultimately become the four-chambered structure with which we are born. There are two upper receiving chambers called the right and left **atria,** and two lower pumping chambers called the right and left **ventricles** (FIGURE 1.1). The right atrium receives venous blood (blood that has delivered **oxygen** and nutrients to cells) from all over the body. The venous blood (contained in two large **veins** called the **superior** and **inferior vena cavae**) passes from the right atrium to the right ventricle through a one-way valve called the tricuspid valve. The right ventricle contracts and pumps this venous blood through another one-way valve, the

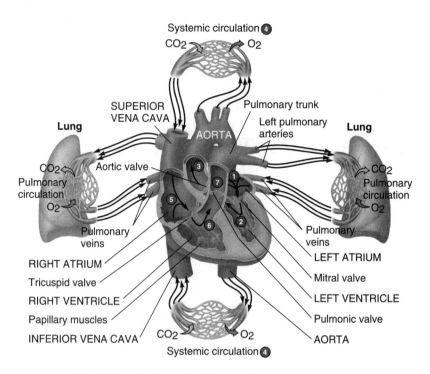

FIGURE 1.1 Blood flowing through the human heart.

pulmonic valve, into the **pulmonary artery.** In the lungs, the pulmonary artery divides into smaller and smaller branches. The smallest branches, called **pulmonary capillaries,** pick up oxygen from and release carbon dioxide into tiny air sacs, called pulmonary alveoli. This enriched blood is then collected into pulmonary veins, which empty into the left atrium. From the left atrium the arterial blood (oxygenated blood) passes through the **mitral valve** into the heart's main pumping chamber, the **left ventricle.** From here, the heart ejects blood through the aortic valve into the **aorta,** the main **artery** from which blood is distributed throughout the body.

The heart is a muscular pump. Like all pumps it needs energy. The heart gets its energy from oxygen in the blood, which is supplied by two little arteries called the **coronary**

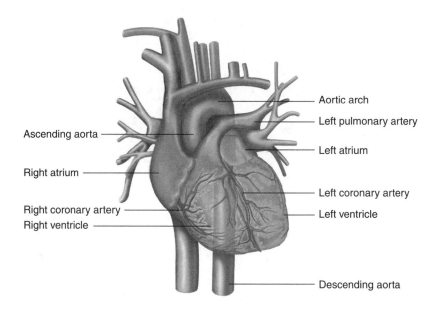

Ascending aorta

Right atrium

Right coronary artery

Right ventricle

Aortic arch

Left pulmonary artery

Left atrium

Left coronary artery

Left ventricle

Descending aorta

FIGURE 1.2 Heart and major arteries.

arteries, the first branches of the aorta (FIGURE 1.2). The right coronary artery supplies most of the right atrium and right ventricle, and usually feeds blood to the inferior surface of the left ventricle. The left coronary artery divides into two major branches called the **left anterior descending artery** and the **left circumflex artery.** These arteries supply the left atrium and most of the left ventricle.

The right ventricle and the pulmonary artery sit in front of the left ventricle and the aorta, just behind the sternum (the breastbone). The left ventricle projects to the left of the sternum so that on a chest x-ray, most of the heart appears to be in the left side of the chest (FIGURE 1.3). Although it is not usually visible on an x-ray, the heart is suspended in a thin sac called the **pericardium.**

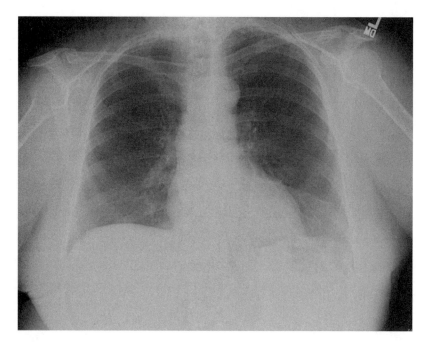

FIGURE 1.3 The heart as viewed by x-ray.

The last bit of information that you need to know in order to understand how the normal heart functions is that the heart contains specialized cells that form tiny electrical currents. You can think of these electrical currents as the heart's batteries. They originate in the heart's **sinus node**, which sits in the right atrium (FIGURE 1.4). The sinus node is a collection of cells that spontaneously depolarize (become electrically excited) an average of 60 times per minute when you are at rest. When you are excited or exercising, the rate raises to over 100 beats per minute. The electrical impulse fans out and travels through the heart along specialized pathways, causing the heart to contract (FIGURE 1.5).

The electrical activity of the heart can be detected and displayed graphically using a test called an electrocardiograph (EKG). An EKG is the most commonly performed cardiac test. A Dutch physiologist named Willem Einthoven

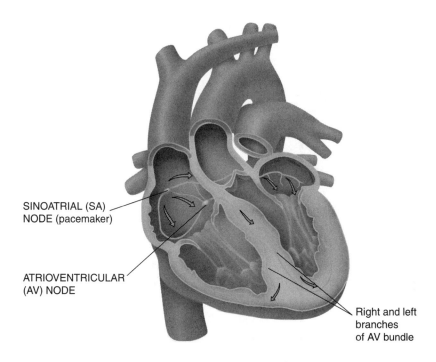

SINOATRIAL (SA)
NODE (pacemaker)

ATRIOVENTRICULAR
(AV) NODE

Right and left
branches
of AV bundle

FIGURE 1.4 The conduction system of the heart. These specialized groups of
cardiac muscle cells initiate an electrical impulse throughout the heart, beginning
in the sinoatrial (SA) node and spreading to the atrioventricular (AV) node. The
AV node then initiates a signal that is conducted through the ventricles.

is credited with inventing the EKG in 1901. In the earliest
prototype, a person had to place his hands and feet in four
buckets of water! In 1924 Einthoven was awarded the Nobel
Prize for this invention.

Over the course of the average life span, the heart pumps
between 4 and 8 liters of blood every minute for more than
75 years. It contracts and relaxes about 2.5 billion times.
If the heart stops for more than 4 or 5 minutes, your brain
suffers irreversible damage and you die. If something injures
the heart and it can't pump enough blood to meet the body's

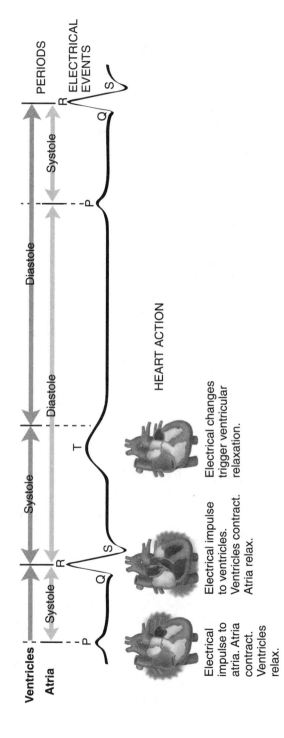

FIGURE 1.5 Events represented by the electrocardiogram. An electrical impulse triggers contraction in the affected muscle tissue. Thus, cardiac muscle contraction occurs after this electrical triggering.

needs, every organ in the body suffers, and a condition called congestive heart failure develops. The potential for such damage is the reason it's vital for you to keep your heart healthy and happy.

Given the obvious differences between men and women, it isn't surprising that there are differences between their hearts. Our understanding of these differences is still growing because, until recently, women weren't included as subjects in scientific studies. The most obvious difference is that, on average, a woman's heart and arteries are smaller than those of a man. This difference has implications in a woman's response to bypass surgery and **angioplasty**. For example, women historically have had higher complication rates when they have angioplasty and a higher risk of dying after bypass surgery. (This is discussed in more detail in Chapters 10 and 11). Women also have higher resting heart rates than men, and their hearts respond differently to exercise. Researchers have discovered that cardiac **risk factors** for women differ in some respects from those established for men. In addition, **coronary artery disease** typically follows a different course in women than it does in men. Therefore, women may benefit less from certain medicines and interventions.

Cardiac risk factors for women differ from those established for men.

Although much remains to be learned, we already have enough knowledge to prevent most **cardiovascular** disease. The main purpose of this book is to get that knowledge out and to motivate people to act on it.

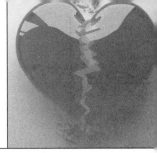

Chapter 2

What Can Go Wrong: The Short Version

In the last chapter, we learned that an adequate blood supply is necessary for the normal functioning of every organ in the body. Arteries deliver blood with its nutrients to every cell in the body. If arteries become narrowed, they are unable to provide the nutrients that cells and organs need to function properly. Hardening of the arteries (**arteriosclerosis**) has occurred for centuries, but it was not until the early twentieth century that this scourge reached epidemic proportions, becoming the leading cause of death in the industrialized world. By the last decade of the twentieth century, **cardiovascular disease (CVD)** had become a leading cause of death in the developing world as well. In fact, about 80% of deaths from CVD now occur in developing countries, and worldwide CVD causes six times more deaths than AIDS.

By the end of the 20th century, cardiovascular disease had become a leading cause of death in both the industrial and developing world.

About a million people in the United States die each year from CVD. Although the mortality rate from cardiovascular disease has been declining in the United States over the last few decades, it has declined less in women than in men.

Arteriosclerosis can take several forms. **Atherosclerosis** is a special kind of arteriosclerosis in which fatty deposits form in the artery's wall. (The word "atherosclerosis" is derived from the Greek word "athera," meaning gruel or porridge, because these fatty deposits appeared soft and lumpy to early pathologists.) The material that builds up in arteries affected by atherosclerosis is called **plaque** (FIGURE 2.1). Plaque is a complex material made up of **cholesterol, smooth muscle cells,** and specialized white blood cells called **macrophages.** The wall of an artery is composed of three layers. The opening through which blood flows is called the **lumen** (FIGURE 2.2). The inner layer of the artery is called the **intima** or **endothelium** and it is the first line of defense protecting the artery from harmful agents that may travel in the blood (like the carbon monoxide given off by cigarette smoke). The second layer which surrounds the intima, called the media, is made up mainly of smooth muscle cells that can contract and relax, allowing the artery to dilate in response to increased demand for blood, or to constrict, for example to prevent **hemorrhage.** When the wall of the artery is damaged, smooth muscle cells migrate into the inner layer and the artery thickens.

A high level of cholesterol in the blood is just one of the factors that can injure the artery wall and make it more permeable. **High blood pressure** is another. **Diabetes,** for reasons that are not fully understood, wreaks havoc with arteries large and small. **Inflammation** also plays a role in

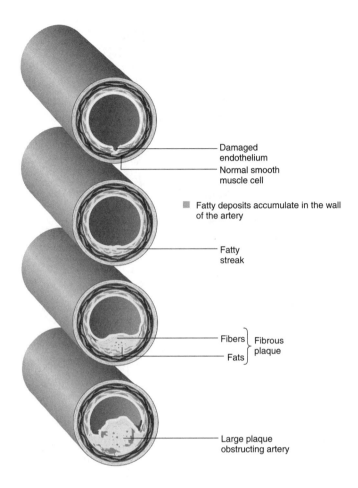

Damaged
endothelium

Normal smooth
muscle cell

■ Fatty deposits accumulate in the wall
of the artery

Fatty
streak

Fibers ⎫ Fibrous
          ⎬ plaque
Fats   ⎭

Large plaque
obstructing artery

FIGURE 2.1 Plaque buildup in coronary arteries.

plaque formation. Many of the chemicals in cigarette smoke directly injure the blood vessel wall and increase the amount of inflammation in arteries throughout the body.

When cholesterol enters the vessel wall, those special white blood cells called macrophages swallow the fats, becoming swollen in the process. Such swollen macrophages are called **foam cells**. The earliest signs of atherosclerosis are **fatty streaks**; they have been found in very young people,

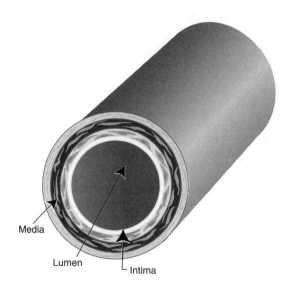

Media

Lumen

Intima

FIGURE 2.2 Cross section of an artery.

and have even been found in the arteries of infants. In fact, a study published in the British medical journal *Lancet* in 1999 demonstrated fatty streaks in fetuses from mothers with high cholesterol levels.

Over time, the plaques can grow and cause progressive narrowing of the arteries. When the arteries supplying the heart become narrowed, people often begin to experience a symptom we call **angina pectoris** (more about this symptom later). Sometimes a plaque can rupture. When this happens, it sets up a chain reaction that often results in a clot that totally blocks blood flow in that artery. If such a blockage occurs in a coronary artery and blood flow is not restored promptly, the heart muscle beyond that clotted artery dies from lack of oxygen (we call this a **myocardial infarction**, what you may know as a **heart attack**).

So how do we prevent this plaque from forming and gumming up our arteries? In the next chapter we'll discuss risk factors for CVD and what to do about them.

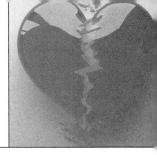

Chapter 3

What Are Risk Factors, and Why Should You Be Concerned about Them?

Framingham, Massachusetts is a town located twenty-five miles west of Boston. Although it may not be famous in the usual sense, to the medical community Framingham reso-nates the way Woodstock does for a rock fan. Much of what we know about risk factors for cardiovascular disease (CVD) derives from studies that were started in Framingham in the late 1940s.

In the early 1900s, animal experiments demonstrated that animals fed a diet high in cholesterol developed plaques in their arteries. At the time, infectious diseases caused most deaths in the United States and elsewhere. Between 1920 and 1940, however, CVD edged out infectious diseases as the number one cause of death in the United States. The National Institutes of Health, the government body that sponsors a large percentage of medical research in the United States, decided in the aftermath of World War II to determine just how common CVD was and to investigate the factors associated with its development.

The Framingham Study was a result of this determination to look into the **epidemiology**—prevalence, incidence, and causation—of CVD. Each one of these types of information is important to determining why, and in whom, a disease is developing or spreading. **Prevalence** is the number of cases of a disease present in a population at a given time. **Incidence** is the rate of occurrence of a disease, that is, how many new cases are diagnosed during a defined time period (usually a year). A **risk factor** is anything that is associated with an increased risk of developing a particular disease. It may be an abnormal laboratory test (such as high blood cholesterol), a behavior (such as smoking, being a couch potato, or overeating), or an inherited trait (such as gender). The Framingham Study was designed to collect information on all of these aspects of epidemiology with the goal of pinpointing risk factors for atherosclerosis—the first step in determining how to prevent and treat CVD.

The study involved 5,209 men and women between the ages of 30 and 62 who were living in Framingham in 1948. Every two years, the subjects of the study had a detailed history taken and underwent a physical examination and various laboratory tests.

The initial results from the Framingham study were published in the 1960s. (The Framingham researchers are now studying the third generation of subjects in this cooperative town, thus continuing to expand our knowledge about CVD.) The results were subsequently confirmed by other large-scale studies conducted here and abroad: age, a family history of heart disease, **cigarette smoking**, elevated cholesterol levels, high blood pressure, diabetes, **obesity**, and physical inactivity are risk factors for the development of CVD.

Some of these risk factors are riskier in women than in men. There are also risk factors that are specific to women. For example, the incidence of coronary heart disease increases in women after **menopause** (whether it occurs naturally or as the result of surgical removal of the uterus and/or the ovaries). Women who have had a hysterectomy before the age of natural menopause have more than twice the risk of coronary disease as premenopausal women of the same age. However, in an article published in the medical journal *Circulation* in 2005, researchers found that among almost 90,000 women who participated in the Women's Health Initiative Observational Study, those who had undergone a hysterectomy (41% of 89,914 women) had more risk factors for developing CVD than women who had not had a hysterectomy (regardless of whether or not the ovaries were removed). Statistical analysis suggested that the hysterectomy itself was not the cause of the increased incidence of heart disease in these women. Rather the researchers believed that the higher incidence of heart disease in women who had hysterectomies was due to their initial adverse risk factor profile.

Another study that looked at the interrelationship of menopause and heart disease was published in the *Journal of the American College of Cardiology* in 2005. The authors used data from the Framingham Study to determine if, rather than being a consequence of menopause, increased cardiovascular risk instead promoted early menopause. In fact, the ovaries have a rich blood supply, and if plaque builds up in the arteries supplying the ovaries this could induce ovarian failure and early menopause.

The study looked only at women who had a natural menopause (as opposed to surgical, or one induced by radiation therapy or medicines). The cardiovascular risk factors that were examined included cholesterol, blood pressure, weight, and the Framingham risk score, which is a method of determining the likelihood of having a coronary event over the next ten years. (The Framingham risk score includes age, total cholesterol, HDL-cholesterol, smoking status, and blood pressure.) Women who used cholesterol lowering or blood pressure lowering medicines were excluded. The study found that women with more cardiac risk factors had an earlier age of menopause. The authors concluded that: "atherosclerosis risk determines age at menopause rather than the reverse."

More recent studies have identified other risk factors for developing CVD. These include an **amino acid** called **homocysteine**, an altered blood fat called **Lp(a)**, a protein that's involved in clot formation called **fibrinogen**, certain markers for inflammation, and, possibly, certain types of infection.

Cigarette smoking causes over 400,000 deaths per year in the United States. What is most appalling is that every one of these deaths is preventable. I tell my patients: "Smoking is just a socially acceptable form of suicide." Even among nonsmokers, multiple studies have now proven that second hand smoke increases the risk of CVD.

Every one of the 400,000 deaths caused by smoking each year is preventable.

Although it's becoming less socially acceptable, about 25% of Americans smoke, and despite advertising campaigns and health education courses in schools the incidence of smoking among teenagers and young adults is rising. About a million young Americans, half of them women, start smoking each year. An estimated one billion people smoke worldwide. In the past few decades, women have started smoking at younger ages and with greater intensity.

There is no more successful crime syndicate in the country than the tobacco industry and its lobbyists. A government truly concerned about health care costs would outlaw the cultivation of tobacco (while compensating tobacco farmers until they could switch to other crops).

Smoking is one of the risk factors that's riskier for women than men. Women who smoke have 1.8 times the relative risk for CVD compared to nonsmokers. The comparable number for men is 1.6. Even before menopause, women who smoke triple their risk of a heart attack compared with nonsmokers.

Women who smoke triple their risk of a heart attack compared with nonsmokers.

In addition to increasing the risk of a heart attack, smoking lowers the age of menopause by about one and one-half to two years. Smokers also have more severe hot flashes during menopause than women who don't smoke. So if you want to age faster, there's no better way to do it than to take up smoking. Smokers have their first heart attack at a younger age than nonsmokers. A study in Denmark found that for women, the median age at first heart attack was 79 in nonsmokers and 60 in smokers. The comparable ages for nonsmoking and smoking men were 71 and 64 respectively. So, not only does smoking lower the age of a first heart attack more for women than men, women smokers, on average, have their first heart attack at a younger age than male smokers. It doesn't take many cigarettes to see the harmful effects of smoking. Even smoking four cigarettes per day was found to double the coronary risk among nurses in the Nurses Health Study. The Nurses Health Study started in 1976 and follows an initial group of 121,700 nurses to evaluate CVD risk factors specifically in women. The study found that the excess risk attributed to smoking decreased by one third within two years of stopping smoking. After more than two years, risk levels for women who stopped smoking fell to the same level as in women who had never smoked.

Smoking is a major contributor to sudden cardiac death in both sexes, but is a particularly striking risk factor in young women. Use of **oral contraceptives** compounds the risk. Currently, women older than age 35 who smoke are advised not to take the birth control pill. Unfortunately, studies have shown that women are less able to overcome addiction to nicotine than men. The reasons for this difference are unknown.

Smoking exerts its harmful effects in many complex ways. Smoking releases carbon monoxide into the blood, which directly injures the artery's wall, thus increasing the influx of cholesterol into the artery. Smoking also raises the level of blood fats called **triglycerides** (more about them later) and lowers the body's level of **high-density lipoprotein (HDL)**, or "good" cholesterol. Nicotine increases pulse rate and blood pressure, and elevated blood pressure is a risk factor for developing of CVD. Additionally, nicotine constricts blood vessels throughout the body, including the skin and the heart. Heavy smokers develop premature wrinkling of the skin because it's chronically starved for oxygen. Moreover, nicotine is more addictive than heroin. Research has shown that 33% of people who smoke one cigarette become addicted to nicotine; only 16% of people who try heroin once become addicted.

Smoking increases the chances for developing **ventricular fibrillation,** an abnormal heart rhythm that's fatal within minutes if it isn't reversed. Smoking makes the blood more apt to clot, and clots are implicated in most heart attacks. In addition to nicotine's constricting effects on blood vessels mentioned earlier, smoking also impairs the ability of arteries to dilate and makes them more likely to go into spasm. It promotes the oxidation of **low-density lipoprotein (LDL)**, the "bad" cholesterol. Oxidized LDL cholesterol is implicated in the growth of plaques. Smoking also increases the blood levels of certain

markers for inflammation—molecules that the body makes when an injury causes an inflammatory reaction.

As if all the above damage isn't enough, there is evidence that heavy smokers have a higher chance of developing diabetes than nonsmokers. A 42% increased risk of developing diabetes was found among women in the Nurses Health Study who smoked 25 or more cigarettes per day. An article in the *International Journal of Epidemiology* in June 2001 reported that among those who smoked two or more packs of cigarettes per day, there was a 45% higher rate of diabetes in men and an astounding 74% higher rate in women compared with nonsmokers. This was a prospective study of more than 275,000 men and more than 434,000 women. Quitting smoking reduced the rate of diabetes in women compared to that of nonsmokers after five years; for men, the rate reduced after ten years.

The damage smoking causes isn't limited to the coronary arteries. Smoking is also a risk factor for developing blockages in the arteries supplying the brain, leading to death and disability from **stroke**. Smoking is a leading contributor to **peripheral vascular disease**, blockages in the arteries supplying the legs that can cause disability and, ultimately, gangrene and amputations. It's also the number one preventable cause of impotence in men. Smokers have a greater risk of developing aortic aneurysms, weakened, ballooned-out areas in the main artery that can rupture and cause death from hemorrhage. In addition to these effects on the cardiovascular system, the poisonous chemicals in cigarette smoke promote the development of various cancers.

Smoking is the number one preventable risk factor for CVD, and it's the number one preventable cause of death in the United States. Stopping cigarette smoking is the most important step that people can take to lower their risk of developing and dying from CVD. Nowadays, most hospitals have programs that use multiple strategies to help people kick their addiction to cigarettes. They use a combination of aids to help with withdrawal, including nicotine patches or gum, drugs such as bupropion (Zyban) and varenicline (Chantix), behavioral modification, and group or individual counseling. If you're a smoker, sign up for one of these programs immediately.

Cholesterol: The Good and the Bad

In 1969, when I finished my internship, the Vietnam War was raging. All young men were subject to the draft. Every male physician stood a good chance of being sent to Vietnam after completing a year of internship. Women were not subject to the draft and, in fact, if a woman had children under the age of eighteen, as I did, she was barred from serving in any branch of the Armed Forces. The United States Public Health Service provided an alternative to Vietnam for a few lucky physicians. These so-called "draft-deferred" positions involved working in underserved areas such as Indian reservations for two years or spending two years engaged in research at the National Institutes of Health (NIH). My then-husband was fortunate enough to get one of these research jobs, and I was offered a non-draft-deferred position at the NIH. My job was in what was then called the National Heart and Lung Institute (NHLI)—now called the National Heart, Lung, and Blood Institute (NHLBI). My boss was Dr. Robert I. Levy. In 1967, Dr. Levy and his colleague Dr. Donald Fredrickson had published a paper on blood fats in the *New England Journal of Medicine* entitled "Fat Transport in Lipoproteins—an integrated approach to mechanism and disorders." Their paper classified an array of diseases involving blood fats. Today, their classification is still used with only minor modifications.

By the time I arrived at the NIH in 1971, the government had decided to sponsor large clinical studies to determine the prevalence of these disorders in the United States and find out if lowering cholesterol in a group of men with high cholesterol would lower their risk of developing signs and symptoms of coronary artery disease (CAD). Although doctors knew from the Framingham Study that high cholesterol was a risk factor, there was no proof that lowering cholesterol also lowered risk. This was an important question to answer because, as we shall see, diet alone cannot lower cholesterol to healthy levels in many people, and the drugs used to lower cholesterol have occasional side effects that range from unpleasant to potentially dangerous.

Dr. Levy named our division the Lipid Research Clinic Program. The Lipid Research Clinic Intervention study provided evidence for the first time that treatment to lower high cholesterol also lowered the incidence of coronary artery disease in men ages 35 to 59 who were initially free of symptoms. This study, like almost all clinical studies at that time, excluded women. So, what do these results mean in relation to cardiovascular health? The following explanation of cholesterol and blood fats will help put these results into perspective.

Cholesterol is a fat—what doctors call a **lipid** (from the Greek "lipos," meaning fat). It's a waxy substance that is found in every cell of the body, where it is an essential component of the cell lining or membrane. It's also required for the synthesis of many hormones as well as substances called bile acids, which are important in the digestion of fats in the intestine.

Cholesterol is insoluble (not dissolvable) in water. Blood is largely water, so in order to be dissolved, cholesterol and other blood fats need to be emulsified or rendered soluble (made dissolvable) in some other fashion. An emulsion—that is, a mixture of two liquids that aren't mutually soluble (think of oil and vinegar in salad dressing)—can be achieved by

shaking, which causes one of the liquids to divide into glob-
ules, called the **discontinuous** phase. The other liquid is then
the **continuous** phase. Milk is another good example of an
emulsion in which the butterfat is the discontinuous phase
and water is the continuous phase. However, evolution must
have decided that vigorous shaking was an inefficient way
to get fats dissolved, and a very efficient system was devised
to transport fat in the blood: the **lipid transport system**. It
evolved to carry otherwise insoluble fats from where they
are made to where they are used. The lipid transport system
works by hooking up fats with proteins called lipoproteins,
which render the fats soluble. **Dyslipidemia** (also known as
dyslipoproteinemia) is a disorder of the lipid transport system.
With this condition, lipid levels are too high or too low.

Lipoproteins are classified according to their density (a
measure of weight per unit of volume). The various types of
lipoproteins include, in order of least to most dense:

- **chylomicrons**
- **very low-density lipoprotein (VLDL)**
- low-density lipoprotein (LDL; also called "bad"
  cholesterol)
- intermediate-density lipoprotein (IDL)
- high-density lipoprotein (HDL; also called "good"
  cholesterol
- Lp(a).

Chylomicrons form in the intestines from fat in the diet.
In the capillaries of muscles and fatty tissue, chylomicrons
are broken down into **free fatty acids**. Free fatty acids are
used by muscle cells for energy or are stored in adipose or
fatty tissue. **Fatty acids** are also taken up by the liver, where
they are repackaged as VLDL. VLDL is then broken down
into IDL. IDL then splits in the liver to form LDL.

Cells in the body can acquire the cholesterol they need
either by making it through a 33-step process or by grabbing

on to particles of LDL by means of something called the LDL receptor, which is located on cell membranes. A mutation in the LDL-receptor gene results in Familial Hypercholesterolemia, a familial disorder in which cholesterol levels are markedly elevated. Familial Hypercholesterolemia is the most common of the genetic dyslipidemias. Individuals affected by it have cholesterol levels in the range of 300 to 500 mg/dL if they're heterozygous (have one mutated gene from one parent) or 500 to 1,000 mg/dL if they're homozygous (have two doses of the mutated gene, one from each parent). Patients with Familial Hypercholesterolemia develop accumulations of cholesterol in the skin, called **xanthoma,** and have premature vascular disease. Those with two mutated genes commonly experience heart attacks in childhood. Those with one mutated gene who go untreated usually develop vascular disease between ages 30 and 50. Despite equivalent cholesterol levels, women with the heterozygous form of the disorder develop signs of vascular disease about ten years later than men do. LDL cholesterol is instrumental in plaque formation and higher levels of LDL cholesterol increase the risk of developing atherosclerosis. However, the level of LDL cholesterol is less predictive of CVD risk in women than it is in men.

HDL, the "good cholesterol," is formed in multiple tissues, including the intestine and the liver. Its metabolism is complex; the details of the process are still being studied. Both the intestine and the liver make the major lipoprotein found in HDL. Across their life span women have, on average, higher levels of HDL cholesterol than men, by about 10 mg/dL. These levels decrease only minimally after menopause.

HDL cholesterol acts as a scavenger. It can actually remove cholesterol from plaques and may also limit the oxidation of LDL cholesterol (remember, it is the oxidized form of LDL that forms part of plaques). For HDL, the higher your level, the better off you are, although recently studies have indicated that some people with very high levels of HDL cholesterol may have

HDL can remove cholesterol from plaques; the higher your HDL level, the better off you are.

an ineffective form of the molecule. An HDL of 60 mg/dL or greater is a negative risk factor—that is, it allows you to subtract one other risk factor from your list.

Multiple studies have shown that a low blood level of HDL is a risk factor for developing atherosclerosis. Most of the time, low HDL cholesterol levels are associated with high levels of triglycerides. This specific combination seems to be particularly risky for women, though we don't presently know why. In women older than age 65, a low HDL level is the most significant lipid predictor of risk.

There are genetic disorders associated with low HDL cholesterol levels. One of these, called Tangier disease after the place where the first case was identified, was what propelled Dr. Levy into the study of lipid disorders. He said that on reading about the disease he decided he wanted to study it, thinking he would get to travel to Africa. Unfortunately, the Tangier in question was an island in the Chesapeake Bay, but by the time he found this out, he was already committed. I'm not sure if he was pulling my leg, but it's an amusing story and a good example of serendipity.

Although Tangier disease is only one of several genetic disorders that can cause abnormal lipid levels, lifestyle and diet also play a role. I tell my patients: "If you pick your parents wisely, you can eat anything you want." This is only partly tongue in cheek. On average, about 85% of your total cholesterol level is determined by your genes; 15% of your total cholesterol level is determined by what you eat. Eating saturated fats (those that are solid at room temperature) raises cholesterol levels more than eating pure cholesterol. Alcohol consumption and regular aerobic exercise raise levels of HDL, as does estrogen, medicines called **statins**, and mega-doses of the vitamin **niacin**. Diets high in carbohydrates raise triglyceride levels. The normal level for triglyceride (and the blood test should be done after a 12-hour fast) is up to 150 mg/dL. Diets very low in fats actually decrease the level of HDL.

Lp(a) is an altered form of LDL cholesterol which will be discussed in greater detail later in this chapter.

Certain diseases can secondarily increase blood lipid levels. These include diabetes, kidney disease, cirrhosis of the liver, obstructive liver disease, and **hypothyroidism** (an underactive thyroid). Various medications have also been shown to raise lipid levels. These include the retroviral drugs used to treat human immunodeficiency virus (HIV) and acquired immunodeficiency syndrome (AIDS), medicines called **beta-blockers** that are used to treat high blood pressure, drugs used to suppress rejection in transplant patients, and some **diuretics** (water pills). Medications that are used to treat dyslipidemias will be discussed in Chapter 9.

High blood pressure is often referred to as the "silent killer." Normal blood pressure is defined as less than 135/85 mm Hg. The upper number is called the systolic pressure, a measurement of the pressure in your arteries when the heart contracts. The lower number is called the diastolic pressure. This is the pressure in your arteries when the heart is relaxing between beats. Blood pressure is measured in millimeters of mercury (mm Hg), the height a column of mercury can be raised to by the pressure in the artery. Optimal blood pressure is 120/80 mm Hg or less.

Approximately 50 million Americans have high blood pressure. The incidence of high blood pressure, also called **hypertension**, increases with age. Hypertension is found in fewer than 20% of those younger than age 40. By age 70, more than 60% of women are hypertensive, and women have a higher prevalence of hypertension than men after age 55.

Population studies have consistently shown that African Americans have about twice the incidence of hypertension as whites. Only about one fourth of people with hypertension receive effective treatment. Untreated hypertension increases the risk of arteriosclerosis, heart attack, congestive heart failure, kidney failure, and stroke. In older women, a 10 mm increase in blood pressure causes a 20% to 30% increase in the risk of heart attack and stroke. Conversely, lowering blood pressure by even one or two points leads to a decrease in risk. Multiple studies over the last few decades have shown conclusively that treating hypertension lowers the incidence of these outcomes. Even people with mild hypertension benefit from treatment.

Untreated hypertension increases the risk of arteriosclerosis, heart attack, congestive heart failure, kidney failure, and stroke.

High blood pressure has been called "the silent killer" because if it's uncomplicated it doesn't cause signs or symptoms. The signs and symptoms that people do associate with high blood pressure, such as headaches, dizziness, or fainting, occur just as commonly in people without hypertension as they do in those with hypertension. There is only one way to determine if you have high blood pressure: Have your doctor or her nurse measure it.

When blood pressure is variable, it's called "labile." A form of labile hypertension that's common in women is so-called "white-coat" hypertension, blood pressure that's elevated in the physician's office, but not elevated in less stressful situations. It's estimated that about 20% to 30% of people have white-coat hypertension. These patients have been shown to have no increased risk of cardiovascular events. Having your blood pressure checked outside of the physician's office will help you determine if you have this problem.

Unlike smoking, hypertension increases cardiovascular risk equally for men and women. However, there is a gender difference in the response to hypertension. Women with hypertension are more than twice as likely as men to develop left ventricular hypertrophy (LVH), abnormal thickening of the muscle in the left ventricle. In the Framingham population, the presence of LVH was associated with an increased risk of cardiovascular complications.

Most hypertension is essential, which is a fancy way of saying we don't know what causes it, but there are also secondary causes. Being overweight is the most common secondary cause of hypertension. Other causes include high salt intake in salt-sensitive individuals, alcohol abuse, cocaine use, and use of oral contraceptives. Women taking oral contraceptives should have their blood pressure measured periodically. If hypertension is detected, oral contraceptives should be discontinued and another form of contraception should be used. Most of the time, blood pressure returns to normal within a few months of stopping oral contraceptives.

Women taking oral contraceptives should have their blood pressure measured periodically.

Your doctor can determine if you should be evaluated for less common secondary causes of HT. Narrowing of an artery supplying the kidney (**renal artery stenosis**) causes about 5 per 1,000 cases of HT, but identifying it is important because successful relief of the obstruction may allow some patients to stop taking blood pressure medication.

Atherosclerosis is the most common cause of this type of HT, called **renovascular hypertension**. Atherosclerotic renal artery narrowing is equally common in elderly men and women, but is more common in men in younger age groups.

Another kind of renal artery stenosis, called **fibromuscular dyplasia**, is the most common cause of renovascular hypertension under the age of 40 and occurs predominantly in women. Renal artery obstruction often causes an abnormal sound in the abdomen, called a **bruit**. Another clue to its presence is failure of blood pressure to respond to intensive medical therapy.

To help gain some perspective on how renal artery stenosis causes hypertension, here is an example from my own professional experience:

Vera, a 55-year-old nurse, had been told by her primary care physician that she had borderline high blood pressure. Although she came to see me complaining of **palpitations**, I was more concerned with her blood pressure, which was quite elevated at 170/104 mm Hg. I prescribed medication for her, but it made her light-headed and did not lower her blood pressure all that much.

I ordered a special kind of **magnetic resonance imaging (MRI)**, a test that uses powerful magnets to construct images of the inside of the body. The MRI showed that one of the renal arteries had signs of fibromuscular dysplasia. Vera had an angioplasty, in which an interventional radiologist used a special balloon-tipped catheter to dilate the narrowed artery. She now has normal blood pressure.

Obesity is another significant contributor to the incidence of hypertension, especially in women. A common measure of obesity is called the Body Mass Index (BMI). It's calculated by dividing a person's weight in kilograms (a kilogram is 2.2 pounds) by his or her height in meters squared. (A meter is 3.3 feet. To square a number you multiply it by itself.) There are several Web sites that calculate your BMI for you if you enter your weight in pounds and height in feet and inches. One such site is *http://www.nhlbisupport.com/bmi/*.

A study in Belgium found that BMI accounted for almost 28% of the variance of systolic blood pressure in women, but only about 10% in men. The Framingham data show that obese women between the ages of 30 and 39 are seven times more likely to develop hypertension than thin women of the same age. Weight loss commonly causes a drop in blood pressure in overweight patients. Lifestyle modification is vital as therapy for both the prevention and treatment of HT. Regular exercise, modest salt restriction, weight loss, and avoidance of alcohol have all been shown to cause modest decreases in blood pressure in persons with hypertension. When these prove insufficient, drug therapy is called for. (See Chapter 9 for more information about drug therapy.)

Diabetes: A Modern Epidemic

Diabetes is a risk factor that is especially dangerous in women. In 1997, the American Diabetes Association published new guidelines for the diagnosis of diabetes. Ordinarily, two hormones made in the pancreas, **insulin** and **glucagon**, regulate the level of glucose (sugar) in the blood within fairly narrow limits. Too low a level of blood glucose (**hypoglycemia**) can cause seizures, coma, and death. Too high a level of glucose (**hyperglycemia**) can cause severe dehydration, build-up of acid, coma, and death. Diabetes is diagnosed on the basis of a blood test. If you have fasted for 8 hours, your blood glucose should be no higher than 100 mg/dL. If your fasting blood glucose is 126 mg/dL or above, you have diabetes. If you have eaten within 8 hours, your blood glucose should be no higher than 140 mg/dL. If your blood glucose measures 200 mg/dL or greater, you have diabetes. If your blood glucose is between these values, you have what is called impaired glucose tolerance, and you may be on your way to developing diabetes.

If you have or are developing diabetes, you're not alone. More than 20 million Americans have diabetes today; this compares with only about 2 million cases of diabetes in the United States in the 1960s. These cases are divided into two main types of diabetes. In **type 1 diabetes** (also called juvenile or insulin-dependent diabetes), a person lacks insulin, causing his or her blood sugar to become very elevated. As indicated by its name, this type of diabetes usually develops during childhood, and it can be caused by genetic, environmental, or immunologic factors. About 90% of all diabetics, however, have what is called **type 2 diabetes**, also known as non-insulin-dependent diabetes and adult onset diabetes. People with type 2 diabetes have higher-than-normal insulin levels, called **hyperinsulinemia**, but their cells are resistant to the actions of insulin. Although genetic factors play a role in the development of type 2 diabetes, lifestyle is also important. Type 2 diabetes is often the result of **obesity**, which has reached epidemic proportions in our population. There is no significant difference in the incidence of diabetes between men and women, but there are marked ethnic differences. African Americans, Hispanics, and Native Americans all have higher rates of diabetes than do white, non-Hispanic Americans.

Atherosclerosis causes about 80% of deaths in diabetics, whether type 1 or 2. About three quarters of these deaths are due to CAD, the rest from strokes or blockages in the arteries supplying blood to the legs.

There is one condition specific to women that's associated with insulin resistance and high blood levels of insulin: polycystic ovary syndrome (PCO). Women with this syndrome have infertility, hirsutism (unwanted hair), and irregular menstrual cycles. The Nurses Health Study II found evidence that women with irregular menstrual cycles or cycles of more than 40 days were twice as likely to develop type 2 diabetes as women with normal cycles. This risk was independent of obesity, which is also common in women with PCO. Women with PCO have higher-than-normal levels of male hormones called androgens. In addition, they tend to have high levels of triglycerides and low levels of HDL. One study has shown that women with PCO have more extensive CAD than women with normal ovaries.

The effects of diabetes on cardiovascular health are particularly harmful in women. In the Framingham population, the incidence of congestive heart failure was increased eightfold in diabetic women ages 35 to 64, as opposed to a fourfold increase in diabetic men. In people older than age 65, diabetes increased the risk of congestive heart failure fourfold in women but only doubled the risk in men. The Framingham Study also showed that patients with type 1 diabetes had a 35% chance of dying from CAD by age 55, compared with an 8% risk in people free of the disease. At any age, a diabetic woman has double the risk of having a heart attack compared to a nondiabetic woman and the same risk as a diabetic man. Having diabetes completely eliminates the advantage that premenopausal women have over men when it comes to CVD.

Diabetics tend to develop diffuse vascular disease that affects medium and small blood vessels. Disease that occurs in the small arteries is called microvascular disease. Microvascular disease that occurs in the small arteries of the eyes, kidneys, and feet can lead to blindness, kidney failure, and gangrene—all well-known and dreaded diabetic complications. Studies have proven that tight control of the blood glucose in diabetics reduces the risk of microvascular complications such as blindness and kidney failure. In 2003, a study published in the *New England Journal of Medicine* proved that tight control of type 2 diabetes not only reduced the risk of microvascular complications, it also reduced the risk of non-fatal heart attacks and strokes and lowered the need for bypass surgery and amputations.

When diabetics develop coronary artery narrowing, they may not experience angina. They can even suffer heart attacks without experiencing pain. This is due to a diabetic complication that affects the nervous system, called diabetic neuropathy. Diabetic neuropathy can cause pain and interfere with the perception of pain.

The Metabolic Syndrome

Other known risk factors tend to cluster in diabetics and pre-diabetics. If someone has three of the five risk factors listed here, he or she is said to have the Metabolic Syndrome. These risk factors include abdominal obesity (a waist measurement of more than 40 inches in men or more than 35 inches in women), an HDL cholesterol below 40 mg/dl in men or below 50 mg/dl in women, a fasting blood sugar over 100 mg/dl, a triglyceride level of 150 mg/dl or more and a blood pressure of 130/85 mmHg or more. The good news is that regular aerobic exercise and weight loss can improve all of these risk factors and has been proven to be of benefit in lowering cardiovascular risk in many studies.

Obesity is not just a fashion issue. Between 1988 and 1994, the Third National Health and Nutrition Examination Survey (NHANES III) conducted studies on a sample of the United States population and concluded that approximately 59% of men and 50% of women between the ages of 20 and 74 had a BMI of 25 or greater. The comparable figures for BMIs of 30 or more were 20% for men and 25% for women. The overall prevalence of obesity in this sample was 22.9%. By the year 2000, the prevalence of obesity increased to 30.5% of the population.

The Fourth National Health and Nutrition Examination Survey (NHANES IV) was conducted between 1999 and 2004. The rates of obesity continued to increase. By 2004, 70.8% of men twenty years of age or older were overweight or obese and 31.1% of them were obese. For women the comparable figures were 61.8% and 33.2%. The NHANES IV data showed that obesity among men over this 6-year period continued to rise, whereas the rate in women seemed to level off. But disturbingly, the rates of obesity among children and adolescents also increased significantly. This has been accompanied by an increase in diabetes and hypertension among young people that bodes ill for future declines in CVD rates.

Normal weight is defined as a BMI of 18.5 to 24.9 kg/m². Overweight is defined as a BMI of 25 kg/m² or greater, and obesity is defined as a BMI of 30 kg/m² or greater. Extreme obesity kicks in at BMIs of 40 kg/m² or more. The table on pages 36 and 37 gives BMIs for various heights and weights. You can see from this table that if you're 5 feet 4 inches tall, you need to weigh less than 145 pounds to be considered of normal weight. On the other hand, if you're 5 feet 7 inches tall, you can weigh 158 pounds and not be overweight. Studies have linked the rise in adult and childhood obesity to sedentary lifestyle (too many hours in front of the TV or computer screen) and a high intake of fast foods, which tend to be loaded with fat calories.

All obesity is not equal. Men and women tend to accumulate fat in different areas. Men tend to store fat in the abdomen; this is called central obesity. Other common terms to describe this are abdominal or visceral obesity. Women tend to store fat in the buttocks and thighs. (Think potbellies versus saddlebags or beer guts versus thunder thighs.) Central obesity is measured by taking the ratio of the waist to the hips. An elevated waist/hip ratio is more common in men than women but in women it appears to be a stronger risk factor for CVD than just an elevated BMI. A waist/hip ratio of greater than 0.8 has been shown to increase coronary risk in women. The presence of central obesity is strongly associated with the metabolic syndrome and its accompanying cluster of risk factors.

Multiple studies have documented the association of obesity and the risk of CVD. The Nurses Health Study found the risk of CAD to be more than three times greater in women with a BMI of 29 kg/m^2 or higher compared with lean women with a BMI of less than 21 kg/m^2. Even women who were mildly overweight, with BMIs between 25 kg/m^2 and 28.9 kg/m^2, had almost twice the risk of coronary disease as lean women. The Framingham Study also confirmed that obesity was an independent risk factor for the development of CVD. Other studies have shown that, in women, central obesity is positively associated with smoking and cycles of weight loss and gain, and negatively associated with physical activity.

In women, central obesity is associated with smoking, cycles of weight loss and gain, and low physical activity.

A report by the Surgeon General in 2001 stated that an estimated 300,000 deaths a year could be attributed to illnesses caused or exacerbated by being overweight or obese. Hypertension is the most common associated complication; the more overweight a person is, the more likely he or she is to have high blood pressure. The prevalence of type 2 diabetes also increases sharply with increasing weight. High blood cholesterol is common among overweight and obese people. Men and women with BMIs of greater than 25 kg/m^2 are twice as likely to have high cholesterol compared to normal weight individuals. The incidence of gall bladder disease and "wear-and-tear" or osteoarthritis is also increased in overweight individuals.

There are racial, socioeconomic, and ethnic differences in the prevalence of obese and overweight individuals. The tendency to be obese or overweight is more common among populations with lower income and educational levels. Among women, obesity is more common in African Americans, Hispanics, and Native Americans. The Bogalusa Heart Study found that the excess obesity in African American females compared with white females appeared at about age 9 and increased with time. Using BMI cutoffs of greater than or equal to 27.3 kg/m² for overweight and greater than or equal to 32.3 kg/m² for severely overweight, this study found that 45.9% and 22.4% of African American women ages 28 to 32 were overweight or severely overweight compared to 18.0% and 8.2% of white women respectively. This disparity is thought to contribute to the fact that African American women have significantly higher rates of hypertension, diabetes, and CVD than their white counterparts. In fact, the death rate from CVD among African American women is 147 per 100,000 compared with 88 per 100,000 for white women and 63 per 100,000 for Hispanic women.

The incidence of overweight and obesity increases with age. As we age, our metabolism slows down and we require fewer calories. So, even if we don't increase the amount we eat, we tend to gain weight. The healthy way to combat this is to exercise. The average American gains 30 pounds between the ages of 25 and 55, and loses an estimated

Fitting exercise into a busy schedule takes discipline and time, but the rewards are incalculable.

Body Mass Index Table

	Normal						Overweight					Obese										Extreme Obesity														
BMI	19	20	21	22	23	24	25	26	27	28	29	30	31	32	33	34	35	36	37	38	39	40	41	42	43	44	45	46	47	48	49	50	51	52	53	54
Height (inches)												Body Weight (pounds)																								
58	91	96	100	105	110	115	119	124	129	134	138	143	148	153	158	162	167	172	177	181	186	191	196	201	205	210	215	220	224	229	234	239	244	248	253	258
59	94	99	104	109	114	119	124	128	133	138	143	148	153	158	163	168	173	178	183	188	193	198	203	208	212	217	222	227	232	237	242	247	252	257	262	267
60	97	102	107	112	118	123	128	133	138	143	148	153	158	163	168	174	179	184	189	194	199	204	209	215	220	225	230	235	240	245	250	255	261	266	271	276
61	100	106	111	116	122	127	132	137	143	148	153	158	164	169	174	180	185	190	195	201	206	211	217	222	227	232	238	243	248	254	259	264	269	275	280	285
62	104	109	115	120	126	131	136	142	147	153	158	164	169	175	180	186	191	196	202	207	213	218	224	229	235	240	246	251	256	262	267	273	278	284	289	295
63	107	113	118	124	130	135	141	146	152	158	163	169	175	180	186	191	197	203	208	214	220	225	231	237	242	248	254	259	265	270	278	282	287	293	299	304
64	110	116	122	128	134	140	145	151	157	163	169	174	180	186	192	197	204	209	215	221	227	232	238	244	250	256	262	267	273	279	285	291	296	302	308	314
65	114	120	126	132	138	144	150	156	162	168	174	180	186	192	198	204	210	216	222	228	234	240	246	252	258	264	270	276	282	288	294	300	306	312	318	324

66	118	124	130	136	142	148	155	161	167	173	179	186	192	198	204	210	216	223	229	235	241	247	253	260	266	272	278	284	291	297	303	309	315	322	328	334
67	121	127	134	140	146	153	159	166	172	178	185	191	198	204	211	217	223	230	236	242	249	255	261	268	274	280	287	293	299	306	312	319	325	331	338	344
68	125	131	138	144	151	158	164	171	177	184	190	197	203	210	216	223	230	236	243	249	256	262	269	276	282	289	295	302	308	315	322	328	335	341	348	354
69	128	135	142	149	155	162	169	176	182	189	196	203	209	216	223	230	236	243	250	257	263	270	277	284	291	297	304	311	318	324	331	338	345	351	358	365
70	132	139	146	153	160	167	174	181	188	195	202	209	216	222	229	236	243	250	257	264	271	278	285	292	299	306	313	320	327	334	341	348	355	362	369	376
71	136	143	150	157	165	172	179	186	193	200	208	215	222	229	236	243	250	257	265	272	279	286	293	301	308	315	322	329	338	343	351	358	365	372	379	386
72	140	147	154	162	169	177	184	191	199	206	213	221	228	235	242	250	257	265	272	279	287	294	302	309	316	324	331	338	346	353	361	368	375	383	390	397
73	144	151	159	166	174	182	189	197	204	212	219	227	235	242	250	257	265	272	280	288	295	302	310	318	325	333	340	348	355	363	371	378	386	393	401	408
74	148	155	163	171	179	186	194	202	210	218	225	233	241	249	256	264	272	280	287	295	303	311	319	326	334	342	350	358	365	373	381	389	396	404	412	420
75	152	160	168	176	184	192	200	208	216	224	232	240	248	256	264	272	279	287	295	303	311	319	327	335	343	351	359	367	375	383	391	399	407	415	423	431
76	156	164	172	180	189	197	205	213	221	230	238	246	254	263	271	279	287	295	304	312	320	328	336	344	353	361	369	377	385	394	402	410	418	426	435	443

Source: Adapted from *Clinical Guidelines on the Identification, Evaluation, and Treatment of Overweight and Obesity in Adults: The Evidence Report*

15 pounds of muscle over the same time span. That is a net gain of 45 pounds of fat! Much of this can be attributed to decreasing levels of physical activity. I tell my patients that if I can fit regular exercise into my busy schedule (and I do), then anyone can. It takes discipline and time, but the rewards are incalculable.

Which brings us to physical activity. A sedentary life-style is the most common cardiovascular risk factor among women in the United States. In 1995, the Centers for Disease Control and Prevention and the American College of Sports Medicine recommended that adults exercise moderately for at least 30 minutes at least five times per week. Despite this recommendation, studies of leisure time physical activity have shown that only about one in four women follows these guidelines. The prevalence of inactivity increases with age; about one half of women older than age 65 report they get no physical exercise at all. Racial, ethnic, and socio-economic disparities are also common. White, non-Hispanic women are more likely to exercise than Hispanic and African American women. Women with higher educational levels and higher income are more likely to exercise than women with less than a high school education and lower income levels.

Regular aerobic exercise lowers blood pressure and blood glucose levels, improves lipid profiles, and lessens insulin resistance.

Regular aerobic exercise has been shown to lower blood pressure, improve lipid profiles, lower blood glucose levels, and lessen insulin resistance. In fact, regular exercise improves insulin sensitivity independent of weight loss. Exercise also has beneficial effects on the clotting system. Regular exercisers are less likely to develop clots, and if clots do occur, the body's ability to dissolve them is enhanced because of exercise. Men and women differ, however, in how effective exercise is. Compared to men, women have less of an increase in HDL cholesterol and less weight loss for similar levels of exercise training.

Unfortunately, women have been underrepresented in the many studies that have assessed the relationship between exercise and CAD. There were 43 such studies between 1950 and 1995, of which only seven included women. Six of the studies analyzed data on women. The results showed that physically active women have about a 60% to 75% lower risk of CAD than inactive women.

The most striking cardiovascular benefits of exercise were seen in a prospective study published in the *Journal of the American Medical Association* in 1989. The study included 3,120 women who were followed for eight years. Their physical fitness level was assessed by walking on a treadmill. The results were astounding. Among the most physically fit women, the age-adjusted rate of death from CVD was 0.8 per 10,000 person-years, compared to 7.4 per 10,000 person-years for the least fit women. To put it in simpler terms, since death rates are higher for older than younger people, the study investigators took age into account by comparing the people in their study only with others of the same age to determine a "raw" death rate for that age group. The death rate for each age group is multiplied by the proportion of study subjects who are in that age group, and the sum of all of these products is the age-adjusted death rate. The rate is expressed in "person-years" to indicate how many such deaths would occur in a given number of people (10,000 people in this case) over the course of a specific number of years (in this instance, one year). Thus, in physically fit women, fewer than one in 10,000 would die of CVD in a year, whereas among the least fit group of women, more than seven in 10,000 would die of CVD—more than *seven times* as many deaths.

A later study showed a decreased incidence of stroke in women with higher activity levels compared with sedentary women, independent of other risk factors. Results from the Nurses Health Study published in 1999 revealed that there was a direct relationship between exercise intensity and reduction in CAD risk. But brisk walking was as beneficial as more vigorous exercise, and sedentary women who started exercising late in life got similar benefits as women who had always been active.

Brisk walking is as beneficial as more vigorous exercise.

The beneficial effects of exercise aren't just limited to the cardiovascular system. A study reported in the *Journal of the American Medical Association* in 2003 reported that women who engaged in regular strenuous physical activity between the ages of 18 and 50 lowered their risk of developing breast cancer. Women who exercise regularly have been shown to experience less severe flushing with menopause than sedentary women. In a Swedish study, only 5% of women who were highly active had severe hot flashes. In women who did little or no exercise, 15% had severe hot flashes. Exercise also lessens the risk of osteoporosis.

There are few guarantees in life, but I tell my patients I can guarantee that if they exercise regularly, they will feel better. This has to do with the ability of exercise to raise the level of beta-endorphins. These morphine-like chemicals are synthesized by the brain. They're our naturally occurring "uppers." They were discovered in the mid-1970s and have been intensively studied ever since. Both exercise and meditation increase endorphin levels. (One of the more interesting studies of endorphins showed that bungee jumping caused a 200% rise in endorphin levels, which was correlated with a feeling of euphoria. But I don't recommend that you go out and take up bungee jumping just to feel euphoric.) Endorphins have been shown to lower blood pressure, inhibit our perception of pain, and suppress appetite. Their levels rise significantly after only 15 minutes of moderate exercise.

I tell my patients I can guarantee that if they exercise regularly, they will feel better.

Studies have shown that people who exercise regularly have a lower incidence of depression than those who don't, and regular exercise has been proven to have a modest effect in the treatment of clinical depression.

Which brings up the question of stress. It's not just the amount of stress in your life that's important. Equally important is how you react to stress. Even mental stress has been shown to increase pulse and blood pressure. Mental stress alone has been shown to cause the coronary arteries to constrict, particularly if they are atherosclerotic. The release of hormones, such as adrenalin, in response to stress can predispose clots to form, and as we have seen, clot formation underlies most heart attacks. If we react to the myriad stresses in life by overeating, smoking, drinking alcohol to excess, or taking illicit drugs, we won't be healthy. If we react to stress by incorporating regular aerobic exercise (and/or meditation) into our daily routine we will be healthier and happier.

If you're a woman older than age 50 (or a man older than age 40) who has been sedentary for a long time, particularly if you have other coronary risk factors, you should speak to your physician before undertaking an exercise program. Your physician may recommend that you have a formal **exercise stress test** before beginning your program to be certain that you can exercise safely.

New and Emerging Risk Factors

Homocysteine (pronounced homo-SIS-teen) is an amino acid. Amino acids are the building blocks of proteins. There is a rare familial disease in which affected individuals have severely elevated blood levels of homocysteine and a very high incidence of premature vascular disease.

Not all studies found an association between elevated levels of homocysteine and CVD. The Atherosclerosis Risk in Communities Study found that elevated homocysteine was a risk factor for women but not for men, but homocysteine was not felt to be an independent risk factor. Currently, neither the American Heart Association nor the American College of Cardiology recommends population-based screening for homocysteine.

Folic acid, also known as folate, is a vitamin that can lower elevated homocysteine levels. Since 1992, folic acid has been added to flour and grain products in the United States, causing about a 10% decrease in homocysteine levels across the population. Daily intake of 400 mg of folic acid reduces homocysteine levels by about 25%. The vitamins B_6 and B_{12} also lower homocysteine levels. Dietary sources of folic acid include fortified breads and cereals, citrus fruits, beans, and tomatoes. Dietary sources of B6 include meat, poultry, fish, vegetables, fruit, and grains. The sources for B_{12} include dairy products, meat, fish, and poultry.

If our blood couldn't clot, we would all bleed to death the first time our skin was nicked. The medical term for a clot is **thrombus,** and a clot that forms in the wrong place or at an inopportune time is called a **thrombosis.** A thrombosis that travels is called an **embolus**. (Sometimes physicians use the term thromboembolus or thromboembolism.) When a clot forms in a vein and inflames it, this is called **thrombophlebitis**. If the clot just sits there and doesn't cause inflammation, it's called phlebothrombosis. A clot that breaks off and travels to the lungs is called a pulmonary embolus.

A cascade of events occurs when blood clots. It's an extremely complex process involving components of the blood vessel wall, plasma proteins, and blood particles called **platelets**. There are certain states in which abnormal clotting is more apt to occur. These are called hypercoagulable states (physicians do love those big words). They occur in people who are laid up in bed after surgery; have cancer, congestive heart failure, or atherosclerotic vascular disease; or are pregnant. In addition, certain medicines increase the likelihood of clotting, and there are familial diseases that cause a hypercoagulable state.

The body has a process to dissolve clots called **thrombolysis**. There are medicines that promote thrombolysis called **thrombolytics** (sometimes called "clot-busters" in the lay press).

Fibrinogen is a plasma protein that's necessary for clotting to occur. It's involved in the final step of clot formation. Fibrinogen levels increase with age, with smoking, and during acute inflammation. High fibrinogen levels are positively associated with obesity, diabetes, and LDL cholesterol, and negatively associated with HDL cholesterol and physical exercise. A class of medicines called fibric acid derivatives reduce fibrinogen levels, as does hormone replacement therapy in women.

At least three population studies, including the Framingham Study, identified fibrinogen as an independent risk factor for CVD. Pooling the results of several studies indicated that people with the highest levels of fibrinogen had almost twice the risk of CVD as those with the lowest levels. Similar to cholesterol, most of our fibrinogen level is determined by our genetic makeup. There is a great deal of variability in fibrinogen levels, and this has limited its usefulness in screening. We have no evidence that lowering fibrinogen reduces risk. One study that looked at lowering fibrinogen by using the fibric acid derivative benzafibrate didn't show a decrease in vascular risk in patients with CAD, despite a 9% reduction in fibrinogen in the treated group.

Lp(a)

Lp(a) is an altered form of LDL cholesterol that is made in the liver. It consists of LDL plus another molecule that is similar to a protein called **plasminogen**. Plasminogen is involved in the system that dissolves clots. There has been some controversy as to whether or not Lp(a) is an independent risk factor for CVD. Some studies have shown an association but others have not. The Framingham Study looked at Lp(a) in 3,103 women who were free of CVD. The women were then followed for an average of 12 years. The Framingham investigators concluded that elevation of Lp(a) was an independent predictor of heart attacks and strokes in women; however some subsequent studies of Lp(a) in women have failed to find such an association. The most recent study that looked at Lp(a) in women found that among over 27,700 healthy women enrolled in the Women's Health Study, those with the highest levels of Lp(a) had about 1.5 times the risk of having a cardiovascular event compared to women with the lowest levels. This association was strongest for women who also had levels of LDL-cholesterol that were above the median level.

In my own practice I have some women with elevated levels of Lp(a), normal levels of cholesterol and triglycerides, and no other risk factors for coronary artery disease (with the exception of a family history) who have developed blockages or even heart attacks at a young age. So I tend to believe the results of the Framingham and Women's Health studies with regard to Lp(a). High doses of the B vitamin niacin and a medicine called fenofibrate lower Lp(a) levels (see Chapter 9).

Whenever tissue is injured, the body reacts with something called the **inflammatory reaction**. It is a defensive response to injury in which the body attempts to heal itself. The cardinal signs of inflammation are pain, swelling, heat, redness, and **disordered function**—that is, the organ or body part can't function as it's supposed to, as in an arthritic joint that can't bend properly or an inflamed muscle that can't lift as much weight as usual. White blood cells are involved, as are multiple proteins, some of which are released into the blood and can be measured as markers of inflammation. We have come to realize that atherosclerosis is an inflammatory process. Even in the earliest stage, that of the fatty streak, white blood cells called **macrophages** play a role. Oxidized LDL cholesterol is thought to be an injuring factor that starts the inflammatory response in the blood vessel wall. Plaques that have more evidence of inflammation are thought to be more prone to rupture and cause heart attacks.

Some of the many markers of inflammation include C-reactive protein (CRP), interleukin, and tumor necrosis factor (TNF). Among these markers, CRP has proven to be the easiest and cheapest to measure. Studies have shown that those with the top 25% of CRP levels have three to four times the relative risk of developing vascular events than those in the lowest quartile. This increased risk was independent of all the other known risk factors. However, most of these data were derived in men. A subsequent study of more than 27,000 women enrolled in the Women's Health Study (who were free of disease at the start of the study) showed that CRP was the strongest predictor of the inflammatory markers. CRP was even a more powerful predictor of future events than the better-known risk factors of high LDL cholesterol and low HDL cholesterol. The relative risk for future cardiovascular events in women in the highest CRP quartile was 4.4 times that of women in the lowest quartile. The investigators concluded that adding a measurement of CRP to the CVD screening process improved the identification of women at risk for future cardiovascular events. It should be noted, though, that CRP levels increase markedly in response to injury or infection; therefore, measuring CRP should be delayed for about 2 to 3 weeks after an acute illness. In fact, the current recommendation is that CRP be measured twice, a few weeks apart, and the average taken to determine the CRP risk number.

Certain bacteria and viruses can cause chronic infections. These infections cause a chronic inflammatory response. Investigators have examined plaques microscopically and identified bacteria and viral particles within them. *Chlamydia* is one species of bacteria that has been found in plaque, but that alone isn't proof that they're causing infection. They may just be innocent bystanders. Prospective studies haven't found that prior exposure to *Chlamydia* or several other bacteria and viruses is associated with increased risk of cardiovascular events. At this point it's not clear that infection plays a role in causing atherosclerosis.

In this chapter we've reviewed the risk factors for CVD. Some of these risk factors we can modify, such as smoking or weight; others we are stuck with, such as age, sex, and our genetic makeup. Yet, the greatest risk factor of all may be ignorance. As cardiologist Pamela Douglas, MD has written, in *A Textbook of Cardiovascular Medicine*,

The greatest risk factor of all may be ignorance.

"Perhaps the most important risk factor for CAD in women is the misperception that coronary artery disease is not a woman's disease—that it's somehow more benign or less important in women than in men." Armed with the knowledge of our risk and our risk factors, we can take the necessary steps to maintain cardiovascular health.

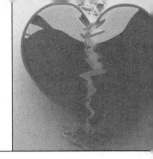

Chapter 4

Know Your Numbers: Prevention Is in Your Control

Scientists have referred to our species as "Homo sapiens," which is Latin for "wise man." I propose a new term to honor the modern American woman: "Femina frenetica." If you're like most of us, you make a whirling dervish look like a lump on a log. You juggle jobs, family, home, and community service. You may take care of everyone around you but neglect to take care of the most important person: yourself. Working yourself into an early grave doesn't do anybody any favors. If you're reading this book, you probably have reason to suspect it's time for some preventive maintenance on the one vehicle you really can't do without: your body. (I'm always astounded by patients who take better care of their cars than themselves. They never miss an oil change or a tune-up. Well, you can trade in your car and get a

If you're reading this book, you probably have reason to suspect it's time for some preventive maintenance on the one vehicle you really can't do without: your body.

new one, but you can't do the same thing with your body.) In this chapter, we'll discuss some important numbers that will help you maintain a healthy heart.

In May 2001, the Expert Panel on Detection, Evaluation, and Treatment of High Blood Cholesterol in Adults published an executive summary of the third report of the National Cholesterol Education Program (NCEP). This panel of eminent scientists wrote that risk assessment was the first step in risk management. So how do you assess your risk?

The panel identified LDL cholesterol as the primary target of therapy. (Remember, LDL is the "bad" cholesterol.) Your optimal level of LDL, however, is based on how many other risk factors you have. The more risk factors you have, the higher your risk of developing atherosclerosis. The panel named five factors that determine your level of risk. The presence of these factors determines the target level of LDL you should have. The major risk factors that modify your LDL goal are listed in the following table.

Risk Factors That Modify Target LDL Levels

- Cigarette smoking
- Hypertension (blood pressure equal to or greater than 140/90 or treatment with blood pressure medication)
- Low HDL cholesterol (less than 40 mg/dl)
- Family history of premature coronary heart disease (coronary heart disease appears in a male first-degree relative younger than age 55 or a female first-degree relative younger than age 65)
- Age (men age 45 or older; women age 55 or older)

Other factors impact your potential for developing coronary heart disease in different ways. For example, diabetes is considered a coronary heart disease risk equivalent. This means that if you have diabetes, you have the same risk of having a coronary event as someone with diagnosed coronary heart disease (CHD)—more than 20% of such people will develop CHD or have a recurrent CHD event within 10 years. HDL cholesterol of 60 mg/dl or higher counts as a "negative" risk factor and allows you to subtract one risk factor from your total. The table below gives your LDL cholesterol goals based on the number of risk factors you have. Remember that diabetes is considered the same as a diagnosis of CHD.

Risk Category—LDL Cholesterol Goals	
Diagnosed with CHD or CHD risk equivalents such as diabetes	less than 100 mg/dl
2 or more risk factors	less than 130 mg/dl
0–1 risk factor	less than 160 mg/dl

In 2004, based on new evidence derived from clinical trials involving people with diagnosed vascular disease a new "optional" LDL-cholesterol goal of less than 70 mg/dl was proposed for people who had both CVD and multiple other risk factors.

Here are some examples of how the presence of risk factors affects LDL cholesterol goals:

Mary is a 52-year-old patient of mine. Her father died of a myocardial infarction (heart attack) when he was 44. Her HDL cholesterol is 45 and her LDL cholesterol is 170 mg/dl; she doesn't smoke or have high blood pressure. Mary has two risk factors for CHD other than LDL cholesterol, so she is assigned an LDL cholesterol goal of less than 130 mg/dl. Leslie, on the other hand, has been a diabetic for ten years.

She's 40 years old and has no other risk factors. Her LDL cholesterol is currently 120 mg/dl, but because she is diabetic (a CHD equivalent) her LDL goal is less than 100 mg/dl. Both of these patients might need to go on medication to reach their LDL goals.

You can total up your risk factors and determine what your LDL goal should be. How do you reach your LDL goal if you are over that number? The first step is to alter your diet to limit your intake of saturated fats and cholesterol.

No diet is going to work if you don't like it. That's my issue with some of the more extreme diets like the very low-fat diet proposed by Dr. Dean Ornish. I never preach anything to my patients that I don't practice myself, and I couldn't stay on such a restricted fat diet for more than an hour or two! Besides, diets that are very low in fat aren't necessarily good for you. Americans have been decreasing the amount of fat in their diet for the last two decades, but the number of overweight and obese people has been skyrocketing. (For an excellent review of the "diet wars," read Gary Taubes' article "What if Fat Doesn't Make You Fat?" which was published in the July 7, 2002 issue of the Sunday *New York Times Magazine*.) The problem with the usual American diet is that it contains too much saturated fat (such as animal fats, coconut oil, and palm oil), not enough nutritious fat (those found in vegetables and fish), and too many simple carbohydrates.

> *No diet is going to work if you don't like it.*

The NCEP recommends the Therapeutic Lifestyle Changes (TLC) Diet for people with unhealthy lipid levels. This diet recommends limiting intake of **trans-fatty acids** (found in margarines, some restaurant foods, snacks, and store-bought pastries) because they raise LDL cholesterol. (More on trans-fats later.)

In addition, the diet recommends that carbohydrates be derived mostly from foods rich in whole grains, fruits, and vegetables. The complete nutrient composition of the TLC diet is given in the table below.

The Nutrient Composition of the TLC Diet	
Nutrient	Recommended Intake
Saturated fat	Less than 7% of total calories
Polyunsaturated fat	Up to 10% of total calories
Monounsaturated fat	Up to 20% of total calories
Total fat	25–35% of total calories
Carbohydrate	50–60% of total calories
Fiber	20–30 grams/day
Protein	Approximately 15% of total calories
Cholesterol	Less than 200 mg/day

Although the table is useful in setting dietary parameters, it isn't particularly helpful when it comes to making food choices. I recommend a time-honored and time-tested diet that is simple, delicious, and healthy: the Mediterranean diet. For a complete explanation of the benefits of this diet, I recommend that you read the book *Low Fat Lies, High Fat Frauds and the Healthiest Diet in the World* co-authored by Kevin Vigilante, MD and Mary Flynn, PhD. As the book points out, studies by Dr. Ancel Keys in the 1950s established that the lowest rates of death from cancer and heart disease were found among the people on the Greek islands of Crete and Corfu (this despite the fact that their diet contained 40% fat). The key was that the fat content of the diet was almost completely made up of olive oil. The book quotes one of Dr. Keys' associates describing the typical diet on Crete: "Olives, cereal grains, pulses (legumes), wild greens, and herbs and fruits together with limited quantities of goat meat and milk, game, and fish have remained the basic Cretan foods for forty centuries...Olives and olive oil contributed significantly to energy intake...Food seemed literally to be 'swimming' in oil."

I'm not saying that your meat selection has to include goat and game. What I am saying is that you should eat meat sparingly—a three-ounce portion (no bigger than the palm of your hand) no more than once or twice per week. (That's if you're healthy and do not have documented CVD—for those of you who have vascular disease it's best to avoid meat completely except on rare occasions. And contrary to popular opinion **chicken is meat**).

You should consume the "fatty" fishes like salmon, trout, sardines, or herring at least twice per week. High consumption of fatty fishes has been linked to a lower incidence of sudden cardiac death. For those with CHD who can't tolerate fish, the American Heart Association has recently endorsed fish oil supplements. In that case, the AHA recommends that you take a one-gram fish oil supplement three times per day.

Your diet should also include eating at least five servings of fruit and vegetables every day. The dried, frozen, and canned varieties by and large are just as nutritious as the fresh. Eat whole grain foods rather than foods made with processed flour, and choose brown rice over white. Snack on nuts and fruit. Limit dairy products to those made with

Once in a while, you may reward yourself with a couple of pieces of dark chocolate.

skim or 1% milk. Once in a while, you may reward yourself with a couple of pieces of dark chocolate. It turns out that chocolate, although it does contain saturated fat, also contains monounsaturated fats (which raise levels of HDL or "good" cholesterol) and flavonoids (nutrients that can lower LDL cholesterol and have cancer-fighting properties). Dark chocolate has also been found to contain compounds that dilate blood vessels and reduce blood pressure.

The Mediterranean diet also works if you have high triglycerides, the other major blood fat. The normal level of triglycerides is up to 150 mg/dl. Levels of 150 mg/dl to 199 mg/dl are considered borderline-high, and levels above 200 mg/dl are elevated. The Mediterranean diet isn't high in carbohydrates, and eating lots of carbohydrates is what raises triglyceride levels. If you're overweight, weight loss is key to getting your triglyceride levels down, so you'll need to limit your calories and increase your exercise to reach your goal.

Calories, however, aren't the only thing we have to worry about. How calories are divided among the major food groups is also an important part of maintaining a healthy diet.

Throughout most of human history, carbohydrates provided the largest source of energy in the diet. Carbohydrates are made up of carbon, hydrogen, and oxygen. Starches and sugars are examples of carbohydrates. The simple sugars (also called monosaccharides) have six carbon molecules that are linked to six molecules of oxygen and twelve molecules of hydrogen. Glucose is an example of a simple sugar; it's an essential food for the brain and its level in the blood is tightly regulated. Double sugars are termed disaccharides. Lactose is a disaccharide found in milk and milk products. Many adults are lactose intolerant, which means they are unable to digest lactose.

Polysaccharides are complex carbohydrates that are made up of long chains of monosaccharides. Polysaccharides can be divided into the starches and the non-starches. Non-starch carbohydrates are the main components of dietary fiber. Dietary fiber can be soluble or insoluble. Insoluble fiber is resistant to digestion and has the beneficial effect of decreasing constipation. Soluble fiber, on the other hand, lowers total and LDL cholesterol levels. Fruits, vegetables, oats, barley, and lentils are good sources of soluble fiber.

High-starch foods include potatoes, wheat, rice, and beans. When starch is digested, it's broken down into simple sugars, which are then absorbed into the blood stream. Some starchy foods are digested more quickly than others. Such foods include most breakfast cereals, bread, and cooked potatoes. They are said to have a high glycemic index (they cause an abrupt spike in blood glucose levels) and should be limited in diabetics. On the other hand, foods containing starches that are digested slowly or have significant amounts of insoluble fiber or fat have a low glycemic index. Carbohydrates yield 4 calories per gram; 28 grams make up one ounce, so one ounce of carbohydrate consumed yields 112 calories.

Proteins are complex molecules that contain amino acids. They're found in every cell in the body. All amino acids contain nitrogen, carbon, hydrogen, and oxygen. Some contain sulfur. About 20 different amino acids are used in the synthesis of human proteins, which consist of 50 to thousands of amino acids. The liver makes some amino acids, but it can't make all of the amino acids that our bodies need. Those that the liver can't make are called essential amino acids. Essential amino acids are found in healthy diets. A protein that contains all of the essential amino acids is called a complete protein; one that lacks one or more essential amino acids is called an incomplete protein. Proteins occur in foods derived from plants and animals. In general, animal protein provides more essential amino acids than plant protein. Vegans who avoid all animal products need to consume different kinds of plant foods to be certain that they're consuming enough of the essential amino acids. Similar to carbohydrates, proteins yield 4 calories per gram. The NCEP recommends that protein intake make up about 15% of daily calories.

Fats (also called lipids) are the body's way of storing energy. When we consume more calories than we burn up, that extra energy is stored in the form of fat in fatty or adipose tissue. Adipose tissue, in addition to being a storage depot, helps maintain a constant body temperature by providing insulation.

The dietary fats important in heart health are divided into saturated fats, monounsaturated fats, and polyunsaturated fats. These distinctions are based on chemical differences among the various fats. A simple rule of thumb is that saturated fats tend to be solid at room temperature, whereas monounsaturated and polyunsaturated fats are liquid at room temperature. Saturated fats are found mainly in fats derived from animal products; two important exceptions are palm oil and coconut oil, which are high in saturated fat.

Monounsaturated fats are found in fish and many plants. Olive oil and canola oil are the best sources of this type of fat. Monounsaturated fats actually *raise* the level of good or HDL cholesterol. Diets that are very restricted in fat actually lower the level of HDL. (All fats raise HDL levels. In fact, saturated fats raise HDL cholesterol most of all, but they also raise LDL cholesterol, so they should be restricted in a heart healthy diet.)

Polyunsaturated fats are found mainly in plants (corn and safflower oil, for example). When people consume diets high in polyunsaturated fats, they lower their LDL levels.

Omega-6 and omega-3 fatty acids are contained in polyunsaturated fats. They're called essential fatty acids because they're essential for life. Unfortunately, the body can't manufacture them; they have to be consumed. Omega-6 fatty acids are used by the body to manufacture certain hormone-like substances. Too much omega-6, however, can worsen inflammation. For example, the inflammation associated with arthritis can worsen if the body has high levels of omega-6 fatty acid. Too much omega-6 fatty acid may also promote the growth of certain hormone-sensitive tumors, such as those that develop in breast and uterine cancer. Omega-6 fatty acids are found in corn, safflower, sunflower and soy oils. The modern American diet is full of corn oil, so most people consume too much of this fatty acid.

Omega-3 fatty acids are the active ingredients in fish oil. They're also found in canola oil, flax seed, hemp seed, walnuts, and green, leafy vegetables. A correct balance between omega-6 and omega-3 fatty acids is essential to good health. We don't yet know the ideal ratio of these oils—those studies are underway—but most Americans need to consume much more omega-3 and much less omega-6.

You may have read about another class of fats: those that contain *trans*-fatty acids. *Trans*-fatty acids occur naturally in small amounts in fats derived from beef and lamb, but the vast majority are produced artificially by food manufacturers. *Trans*-fatty acids are formed by adding hydrogen to polyunsaturated fats. They're solid at room temperature and are used to prolong the shelf life of baked goods and other products, such as peanut butter. Margarine is an example of a manufactured food that contains *trans*-fatty acids. Unfortunately *trans*-fatty acids raise LDL and lower HDL cholesterol. *Trans*-fatty acids also interfere with the metabolism of essential fatty acids. They're one of the reasons I tell my patients that if they really are serious about heart health, they won't eat a pastry they didn't bake themselves, using a margarine like Smart Balance that doesn't contain any trans fats. Holland has actually banned the use of *trans*-fatty acids. Some dieticians and physicians are calling on the Food and Drug Administration to do the same. An important point to remember about trans-fats is that Congress, at the behest of various lobbyists, allowed food companies to put on their products that they contained 0 trans-fats, if the amount of trans-fats *per serving* was less than 500 mg. But most of us don't limit ourselves to one serving. It's therefore important that you read food labels carefully. If "partially hydrogenated vegetable oil" is listed among the ingredients, don't buy that product because "partially hydrogenated vegetable oil" is another term for trans-fat.

Plant stanol esters (PSEs) are another manufactured food product that have been in the news. Plants contain chemicals called sterols and stanols that resemble cholesterol chemically. (Remember, cholesterol is found only in animal products.) The plant stanols are combined with canola oil to form PSEs. PSEs lower cholesterol levels by blocking the absorption of cholesterol from the gut. Consuming 3.4 grams/day of PSEs lowers cholesterol levels about 10% and LDL levels about 14%. Benecol contains PSEs and has FDA approval to claim that it lowers cholesterol. Unfortunately the product is quite expensive, costing more than $5.00 for an eight-ounce tub.

In 1996, the FDA approved a fat substitute called Olestra. Olestra's structure is similar to triglyceride, but it can't be digested or absorbed. It's only approved for use in snack foods such as potato chips and crackers. However, Olestra can interfere with the absorption of the fat-soluble vitamins A, D, E, and K, so these vitamins must be added to any foods made with Olestra. The most common side effects from eating foods containing Olestra are loose stools and cramping.

Olestra has also been shown to lower levels of carotene. Carotene is one of a class of molecules called phytochemicals. These plant-produced molecules are antioxidants. Antioxidants help prevent oxidation, a chemical reaction in which oxygen is joined to another molecule. The most common example of oxidation is rust, which results when iron combines with oxygen. Although we need oxygen to survive, too much oxidation is damaging to cells. We're still learning about the role of antioxidants in health and disease, but it's likely that diets high in plant phytochemicals, such as the Mediterranean diet, offer protection against heart disease and cancer because of the high intake of naturally occurring antioxidants. Therefore, it isn't good to consume a food additive such as Olestra that lowers levels of an important antioxidant. Overall, we don't know about the long-term safety of fat substitutes.

Most Americans consume far too much fat, and particularly far too much saturated fat.

Just as there are essential amino acids, there are essential fatty acids, so you need some fat in the diet to survive. The problem is that most Americans consume far too much fat, and particularly far too much saturated fat. Some of us get 50% to 60% of our total daily calories in the form of fat. Following the Mediterranean diet, however, will insure that you're getting the right amount of the right kind of fat.

No discussion of prevention is complete without a word about exercise. We've already noted that the number of overweight and obese individuals has reached epidemic proportions in the United States and much of the industrialized world. This isn't surprising when we compare how our species evolved with how we live today. For hundreds of thousands of years our ancestors lived in caves (at least, the lucky ones did). At that time agriculture and the domestication of animals had not yet been invented. Our ancestors were hunter-gatherers. They either gathered nuts, berries, and wild grains or hunted animals to sustain themselves. So, if our early ancestors wanted to eat, they had to get off their butts and walk until they found or killed something edible. We didn't evolve as a sedentary race. We evolved as a race that spent a good part of the day walking around looking for our next meal. We ate everything edible we could get our hands on, but we expended a lot energy finding that food in the first place. Back then, our ability to store extra calories in the form of fat was crucial because food supplies were always iffy. When food was nowhere to be found, such fat storage allowed our ancestors to survive weeks without starving to death. Being efficient converters of extra calories into fat gave us an evolutionary advantage. But until the modern era, if we didn't keep moving, we just didn't eat. (Even after the domestication of plants and animals about 5,000 years ago, a fair amount of physical work was still required to produce what we ate.)

Nowadays, not only do most people spend most of their time doing nothing more strenuous than poking a computer keyboard, they consume a diet that's far richer in fat than that consumed by our hunter-gatherer ancestors. We take in thousands of calories a day, but we burn up relatively few in the course of our usual daily activities. The result? Obesity runs rampant and contributes to the toll taken by cardiovascular disease.

It's a simple fact of life that calories consumed have to equal calories used if we want our weight to be stable. Now for some discouraging news: You have to burn 3,500 more calories than you take in to lose one pound. At rest, an average-size woman burns about one calorie per minute. Walking at the brisk pace of 4 MPH (which equals 15 minutes per mile) burns 4 calories a minute. Jogging at a rate of 7.5 MPH (8 minutes per mile) burns about 10 calories a minute. To lose weight, we have to limit calories and increase exercise.

> *It's a simple fact of life: to lose weight, we have to limit calories and increase exercise.*

It's beyond the scope of this book to go into the debate over the causes of obesity. It's true that the regulation of appetite is a complex phenomenon that involves the nervous and endocrine systems, and our metabolic rate, the rate at which we burn up calories, is influenced by our genetic makeup. Despite this information, the bottom line is that no one gains weight unless calories taken in exceed the calories burned. Everyone loses weight on starvation diets. (We've all seen pictures of people in concentration camps or famine victims.) Everyone gains weight when they consume more calories than they burn up. It's really as simple as that. This isn't to imply that I don't have sympathy for people who are struggling with being overweight or obese. I have tremendous sympathy for them, but nothing positive is achieved by not facing facts. If you're in denial about the amount of food you consume or how much exercise you get, you're unlikely to achieve your goals.

If you're serious about maintaining a healthy circulatory system, and you're the typical American who consumes too many of the wrong kinds of food and gets little or no exercise, you must commit to some major lifestyle changes.

The NCEP panel recommends that people engage in moderate exercise each day to burn up about 200 calories. The safest, most physiologic way to do this is to walk at a 15 minute per mile pace for 50 minutes a day. If you can't take that long a walk all at once, divide it up into whatever will fit your schedule. You might walk 10 minutes before work, 30 minutes over your lunch breaks and 10 minutes after work. It really isn't that hard. If everyone adopted this exercise prescription and limited their portion sizes, the current epidemic of obesity would vanish.

When you get right down to it, preventing cardiovascular disease is extremely simple...and extremely difficult. If you smoke, **STOP!** If your weight, cholesterol, blood glucose, or blood pressure is high, **GET IT DOWN!** Get at least 50 minutes of **AEROBIC EXERCISE** most days of the week. Also, pick your parents wisely. (If you figure out a way to do this, I can guarantee that the Nobel Prize committee will be giving you a call.) Joking aside, finding the will and the time to make these healthy changes is a tremendous challenge. At the Women's Cardiac Center at the Miriam Hospital, we urge all of our patients with risk factors to consult one of our behavioral medicine specialists for help in making these crucial lifestyle choices. In Chapter 9, I'll discuss the medications your physician will prescribe if, despite these changes, your cholesterol or blood pressure is still too high for heart health.

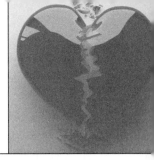

Chapter 5

"I'm Out of Estrogen and I Have a Gun!": The Great Estrogen Controversy

The title of this chapter is a quote from a bumper sticker that I see on a car in the hospital parking lot. I haven't met the driver yet, but I'm amused by this sticker in part because of the derivation of the word estrogen. (Having studied Latin for four years in high school, I am something of a word freak.) The term estrogen (one of the female sex hormones) is derived from the Latin word "estrus," which means "frenzy." Estrus refers to the period of heightened sexual arousal and receptivity that occurs in mammals (except humans) on a recurring basis during their reproductive years. It's what we mean when we say an animal is "in heat." (Human females have a menstrual cycle and are, theoretically, always sexually receptive—except when they have a headache.) So, based on the Latin root of the word estrogen, you can see that if you're out of estrogen, you would actually be less likely to be frenzied and less likely to use a gun.

~

As mentioned in an earlier chapter, menopause is the only cardiovascular risk factor that's specific to women. Premenopausal women have a lower incidence of cardiovascular disease (CVD) than men. By age 75, however, men and women have an equal risk of CVD. Because of the greater number of women in older age groups, more women than men die of CVD each year.

The ovaries produce male hormones (androgens) and female hormones (estrogens and progestins) until menopause. After menopause, production gradually decreases. Estrogen can also be synthesized in other organs, including the adrenal gland and fatty tissue.

One of the most commonly prescribed forms of estrogen is called Premarin. The drug was named Premarin because it was first derived from the urine of pregnant mares. Horses and other members of the genus *Equus* are champion estrogen producers. Surprisingly, the only animals that produce more estrogen per day than mares are stallions, which secrete more estrogen than any other creature that has been studied.

Data from the Framingham Study and other studies made it apparent that premenopausal women have a low risk of CVD compared to men in the same age group. Scientists theorized that estrogen was the cause of this discrepancy and decided to study whether treatment with estrogen had a protective effect. What I find interesting, though, is that the Framingham Study also showed that women who had premature menopause because of hysterectomy had an increased risk of CVD compared with women of the same age who weren't menopausal *whether or not the ovaries were removed or left behind.* It seemed that an intact, bleeding uterus was what protected women from developing CVD prematurely, not whether they had functioning ovaries. This fact was overlooked, however, in the push to see if there was a pill that would protect menopausal woman from CVD.

This particular situation is an example of the problems that can arise in science when we assume that men are the "norm." If scientists studying CVD considered that women were the "norm," they would believe that it would be abnormal for CVD to occur as early as it does in men. They would look for something about men that would make them prone to what would be considered premature atherosclerosis. As a result, scientists might think that the higher levels of testosterone in men were the culprit. Scientists might then want to treat men with drugs that blocked testosterone to see if they could delay the onset of atherosclerosis to an age similar to that of women. Although this scenario isn't likely to occur in reality, it does illustrate my point that assuming men are "the norm" can lead to problems.

The first study that tested the hypothesis that estrogen could protect against heart disease was actually done in men. The study took place in the 1960s and was called the Coronary Drug Project. During the study, estrogens were given to male subjects to see if treatment with the female hormone would lower the risks of cardiac events in men with established coronary artery disease (CAD). At that time, there were only a few drugs available to lower cholesterol, and estrogen was known to have such an effect. Unfortunately, the results with estrogen were uniformly negative. The men treated with estrogen had an *increased* incidence of cardiac events. Not only that, they developed painful breast enlargement. Although men may enjoy large breasts in a woman, they found growing a set of their own unacceptable!

Many observational studies showed that postmenopausal women on **estrogen replacement therapy (ERT)** had a lower chance of dying from CVD than women who weren't on ERT. When the results of more than 30 of these studies were pooled, it appeared that postmenopausal women on ERT had about a 50% reduction in their risk of CVD.

Estrogen has several known beneficial effects that could explain the lower incidence of CVD in premenopausal women. Estrogen lowers LDL cholesterol and raises HDL cholesterol. It decreases the oxidation of LDL and decreases the uptake of cholesterol into the blood vessel wall. Estrogen also dilates normal blood vessels. Lack of estrogen is associated with a decrease in blood vessel elasticity.

Despite the above benefits of estrogen, its use in post-menopausal women who have an intact uterus is known to increase the risk of uterine cancer. This risk can be avoided by taking another ovarian hormone called **progesterone**. (Another term for progesterone and similar hormones is progestin.) Women taking both estrogen and progesterone are said to be receiving hormone replacement therapy (HRT).

The observational studies that appeared to show a benefit of postmenopausal ERT had some important limitations. A brief discussion of epidemiologic research and how it's carried out will help clarify why there was so much controversy about HRT.

As was noted in Chapter 3, epidemiology is the branch of medicine that studies disease prevalence (the number of cases of a disease that are present in a population at a given time), incidence (how many cases of the disease are diagnosed during a defined time period—usually a year), and causation. Epidemiologic studies can be either experimental or observational. In experimental studies (also called clinical trials) some form of intervention is performed on the participants. The participants are then followed over time to predetermined endpoints (such as death or the occurrence of a heart attack). They are assigned to one of two groups: the treatment group or the placebo (control) group. In the most rigorous studies, there are no important differences between the treatment and control groups except that one group gets the treatment medicine and the other gets a dummy medicine called a placebo. In this situation, neither the investigators nor the participants know which medicine an individual is receiving. This type of study is referred to as a randomized, double-blind, placebo-controlled study. Results from such trials are believed to provide the most scientific information because, ideally, there is no bias in assigning participants to treatment or placebo, the participants are followed prospectively, and the endpoints are determined without knowledge of the treatment status of the participants.

On the other hand, no intervention takes place in observational studies. In this type of study, a population is studied over time. For example, the outcomes for women taking ERT are compared with the outcomes for women who aren't taking ERT. A major problem with this type of study is that they may be biased by what's termed "self-selection." In other words, women who elect to take ERT may be a healthier subset of women than those who don't elect this treatment. They may have fewer risk factors and receive more preventive care than women who don't take ERT.

Two important types of clinical trials (experimental studies) are called primary prevention and secondary prevention trials. A primary prevention trial is one in which the participants are free of the disease being studied when they enter the trial. One half of the participants are given a medicine (or other intervention) that hopefully will prevent or lower the incidence of the disease. The other half of the participants are given a placebo. The participants are followed over time to see if people in the treated group develop less angina, heart attacks, or death (in the case of coronary artery disease trials), than the people in the placebo group. In secondary prevention trials, all of the participants have already been diagnosed with the disease being studied. The investigators treat half of the participants with a medicine and half with a placebo. The outcomes of the two groups are measured prospectively.

In 1995, researchers presented the results of a double-blind controlled study of the effect of hormone replacement on cardiac risk factors in 875 healthy postmenopausal women ages 45 to 64. Called the Postmenopausal Estrogen/ Progestin Interventions (PEPI) Trial, the study looked at the effect of HRT on HDL cholesterol, systolic blood pressure, insulin, and fibrinogen (a protein involved in the formation of blood clots). The investigators found that estrogen alone or in combination with a progestin improved lipid profiles and lowered fibrinogen levels without changing insulin levels in response to a glucose challenge. (In a glucose challenge, a person is given a measured amount of glucose and then their insulin levels are measured over a pre-determined period of time.) These results made it seem likely that treating those women at the highest risk for CVD—those past menopause—would lower their risk of developing CVD or lower the incidence of new cardiovascular events in women who already had heart disease. The NIH subsequently sponsored a primary prevention trial, the Women's Health Initiative (WHI), and a secondary prevention trial, the Heart and Estrogen/Progestin Replacement Study (HERS).

HERS was the only randomized, double-blind controlled study of secondary prevention in women with CAD treated with HRT. The results of this study, published in 1998 in the *Journal of the American Medical Association*, were unexpected. The objective of the trial was to determine if therapy with estrogen and progestin altered the risk of coronary heart disease events in women with established CAD. The trial consisted of 2,763 postmenopausal women younger than age 80 who hadn't previously had a hysterectomy. Half of the participants were treated with estrogen and a progestin; half received a placebo. The average age of the participants was 67.

The primary outcomes that were measured were the occurrence of a nonfatal heart attack or death due to CHD. Secondary outcomes were also looked at, including whether a participant needed bypass surgery or angioplasty and whether a participant had unstable angina, congestive heart failure, resuscitated cardiac arrest, stroke (or its precursor, transient ischemic attack), and peripheral arterial disease. Overall, after four years of follow-up, there were no significant differences between the treated and control groups in any of the primary or secondary outcomes. In fact, in the first year of the trial there were more adverse cardiac events in the treated group than in the control group. There were 17 deaths and 42 nonfatal heart attacks in the treated group in the first year compared to 11 deaths and 29 nonfatal heart attacks in the control group. This was a highly significant difference; however, in subsequent years of follow-up there seemed to be a trend toward lowered risk in the treated group, but this trend didn't achieve what physicians call "statistical significance." This means the results weren't significant enough to be attributable to anything other than chance. In the fourth and fifth years of the study there were 49 cardiac events in the placebo group compared to 33 events in the treated group. Because of this trend, the study participants were asked to stay on their assigned treatment and were followed for a longer time.

The results of this prolonged follow-up were published in the July 3, 2002 issue of *The Journal of the American Medical Association*. The study showed that after more than six years the lower rates of coronary heart disease that appeared during the fourth and fifth didn't persist. The researchers concluded from

The study found that once a woman was diagnosed with coronary heart disease, there was no benefit to treating her with hormone replacement therapy.

this study that "after 6.8 years, hormone therapy did not reduce risk of cardiovascular events in women with CHD. Postmenopausal hormone therapy should not be used to reduce risk for CHD in women with CHD." Simply stated, once a woman was diagnosed with CHD there was no benefit to treating her with HRT.

In addition to the results described above, the HERS trial found that women on HRT had a higher incidence of gall bladder disease, venous clots, and pulmonary emboli (clots that break off and travel to the lung from another part of the body). Also, there was no evidence to suggest that HRT increased the incidence of cancer.

The HERS results were disappointing to many physicians and women (not to mention drug companies) because it was hoped that by taking HRT women could maintain the cardiovascular health advantage they have over men in the premenopausal years. It must be noted, though, that HERS had some limitations. For example, it's been suggested that progestins may *oppose* the heart-protecting effects of estrogen. In fact, the progestin used in HERS was shown in the PEPI trial to blunt the estrogen-associated increase in HDL more than other progesterone preparations. Also, HERS didn't evaluate the effect of estrogen alone, and the expected number of cardiac events was smaller than expected. These factors made finding a beneficial result of HRT less likely.

Taking the limitations of HERS into consideration, the researchers theorized that there might be a subgroup of women who are more likely to experience clotting side effects from estrogen. These women might account for the increased number of cardiovascular events in the first year of the study. Unfortunately, there is no way to identify these more susceptible women.

~

As disappointing as the HERS results were, many physicians and patients continued to hope that the WHI study would show that HRT would lower the risk of subsequent cardiac events in postmenopausal women who were free of CVD. Unfortunately, more bad news was in the offing.

The Women's Health Initiative Hormone study was the largest randomized trial of postmenopausal hormone replacement therapy ever undertaken. At the time these studies were designed in 1991–1992, there was widespread belief that HRT after menopause would protect women from developing CVD, even though no randomized, placebo-controlled trials had been performed. In fact, one of the principal investigators told me that she fielded many angry calls from physicians of patients who were interested in taking part in the study, demanding to know how she could justify the fact that half the women in the study would be on placebo, since they "knew" that HRT was beneficial in preventing heart disease.

Despite the opposition of many physicians, however, the study was successful in enrolling tens of thousands of women. They were divided into two groups, depending on whether or not they had had a hysterectomy. (As was mentioned earlier, giving women with an intact uterus unopposed estrogen after menopause increases her risk of uterine cancer. That risk can be abolished by treating with progesterone.) The women who had had a hysterectomy were randomized to two groups. One received a standard dose of Premarin, 0.625 mg per day, and the other received a placebo. There were 10,739 women in this estrogen-only arm, ranging in age from 50 to 79, with an average age of 64.

There were 16.608 women in the WHI Hormone study who had not had a hysterectomy. Their age range was from 50 to 79 years and their average age was 63 years. They were randomized into two groups, one receiving Prempro, the most commonly prescribed HRT in this country (containing 0.625 mg of Premarin and 2.5 mg of medroxyprogesterone acetate) and the other receiving placebo.

An article in the July 17, 2002 issue of the *Journal of the American Medical Association* reported that researchers had stopped the estrogen with progesterone portion of the WHI cardiovascular study prematurely. The trial was planned to last eight and one-half years, but on May 21, 2002, after an average of about five years of follow-up, the trial was stopped. The data and safety monitoring board recommended stopping the trial prematurely because the treatment demonstrated no beneficial effect on CHD events and there was a significantly higher incidence of invasive breast cancer in the women receiving Prempro. In fact, the treated women had more strokes, more pulmonary emboli, and more heart attacks than the women on the placebo. There were fewer cases of colon cancer and hip fractures in the women on HRT, but these benefits were outweighed by the adverse breast cancer and CHD risks. Overall, mortality rates didn't differ between the treated and placebo groups.

Although the absolute number of adverse events in the WHI study was small, there was still cause for concern. For every 10,000 patient years (a "patient year" means following a patient for one year. So 10,000 patient years means following 10,000 patients for one year) of treatment with HRT, there were seven more cardiac events, eight more instances of invasive breast cancers, eight more instances of pulmonary emboli, and eight more cases of stroke. When you consider that more than 22 million prescriptions for Prempro were written in 2000, this translates into 17,600 extra cases of breast cancer, stroke, and pulmonary embolus, and 15,400 *extra* cardiac events. The data and safety monitoring board therefore recommended stopping the estrogen plus progesterone arm of the WHI trial.

For many years doctors thought that the breast tumors that occurred in women taking HRT were less aggressive and were diagnosed earlier than those in women who didn't take HRT. This theory was yet another misconception that was exposed by the WHI study. The WHI study found that there were 245 total cases of breast cancer in women receiving Prempro and 185 cases of breast cancer in women receiving placebo. Of these, 199 of the cancer cases were classified as invasive in the HRT group; 150 were classified as invasive in the placebo group. The invasive breast cancers in the women on HRT were larger and were at a more advanced stage than those found in the women on placebo. In addition, in every year of the study, more women in the treated group had abnormal mammograms than women in the placebo group. It was concluded that treatment with estrogen and progesterone in postmenopausal women may stimulate breast cancer growth and interfere with breast cancer diagnosis.

Since the WHI study was stopped, more bad news has appeared in the press about treating postmenopausal women with estrogen and progesterone. When the WHI investigators looked at dementia in the women in the trial they found that women older than age 65 who received HRT had more than twice the risk of developing probable dementia over the course of the study than women in the placebo group.

The estrogen-only arm of the WHI Hormone study was continued even after the premature ending of the trial that randomized women to either Prempro or placebo. Then, in February 2004, after reviewing data through November 2003, the estrogen-only arm of the study was also stopped prematurely. The researchers found that in this group of women the risk of stroke was increased, and the incidence of coronary heart disease events was not significantly reduced over an average of 6.8 years of treatment. Unlike what was found with combination HRT, the women treated with estrogen only did not have an increase in breast cancer risk; they in fact had a small but statistically insignificant decrease in breast cancer risk.

These results from both arms of the WHI study did not however end the controversy over the use of hormone replacement therapy after menopause. Some scientists criticized the design of the studies, pointing out that in real life it would be unusual to start a woman on HRT or ERT in her sixties or seventies, presumably many years after the menopause. Indeed, on further analysis of the data, there was a trend towards reduction in CHD events in women in the two studies who began therapy less than 10 years after menopause, compared to women who began therapy at a more distant point from the time of menopause, but this trend did not achieve statistical significance (meaning that it might have occurred by chance). Stroke risk was increased in women who took hormones after menopause, even in younger women, and regardless of the time that had elapsed from menopause.

There are women who experience great distress from hot flashes and night sweats around the time of menopause. These symptoms respond better to hormone replacement therapy than to any over-the-counter medicines or herbal remedies. In 2007 the North American Menopause Society published a position paper on "Estrogen and progestogen use in peri- and postmenopausal women." The authors noted that the effects of either estrogen alone or estrogen plus progesterone on the risk of CHD in women with "moderate to severe menopause symptoms" have not been established by randomized controlled trials, since such women (that is those with severe menopause symptoms) were not enrolled in either HERS or the WHI Hormone study. The authors of the position paper therefore wrote that that "extended use of the lowest effective dose" of hormones was "acceptable" provided that the woman is "well aware of the potential risks and benefits and that there is clinical supervision."

Finally, in 2007 a panel of experts published revised "Evidence-Based Guidelines for Cardiovascular Disease Prevention in Women" in *Circulation*, the journal of the American Heart Association. Based on the available data the panel wrote that: "hormone therapy...should not be used for the primary or secondary prevention of CVD."

For women who want to help prevent or treat osteoporosis (brittle bones), there are other medicines that are effective. The class of medicines called biphosphonates work by inhibiting the breakdown of bone. Two medicines of this class are risedronate (Actonel) and alendronate (Fosamax).

Another class of medicines, called the selective estrogen receptor modulators (SERM) have also been shown to prevent osteoporosis. The first drug in this SERM class was tamoxifen (Nolvadex); tamoxifen is useful in the treatment of certain breast cancers. Tamoxifen lowers total cholesterol and Lp(a) levels and raises HDL cholesterol levels. It is not prescribed for osteoporosis prevention, but a different SERM, raloxifene (Evista) has been approved for this use. Raloxifene also lowers LDL cholesterol and Lp(a) levels but has no effect on HDL cholesterol levels. In 2002, the results of a study of more than 7,700 women who were treated with either raloxifene or placebo were published in the *Journal of the American Medical Association*. The study looked at the effect of raloxifene on cardiovascular events in postmenopausal women with osteoporosis. Overall there was no significant difference between the two groups in the number of coronary events or strokes. However, in a subset of more than a thousand women who were at increased cardiovascular risk, those treated with raloxifene had a 40% reduction in cardiovascular events. Like estrogen itself, SERMs have been associated with an increased risk of clots in veins. They also cause hot flashes in some women.

Because of the observation that women at high risk for CVD appeared to lower that risk when treated with raloxifene for osteoporosis in the study mentioned above, a larger study, Raloxifene Use for The Heart (RUTH) was undertaken to see if treatment with raloxifene in women who either had CHD, or had multiple risk factors for CHD would lower the risk of having a coronary event such as heart attack, hospitalization for an acute coronary syndrome (this is the diagnosis given to people who suffer worsening episodes of angina or small heart attacks), or death from CHD. The study also undertook to answer the question as to whether or not raloxifene would lower the risk of breast cancer in these women. The study group comprised 10,001 postmenopausal women with a mean age of 67.5 years who were randomly assigned to treatment with either placebo or 60 mg/day of raloxifene. The results of the study were published in the *New England Journal of Medicine* in July 2006. While raloxifene had no effect on the likelihood of a coronary event, it did significantly decrease the risk of invasive breast cancer (40 occurred in women on raloxifene compared to 70 in women on placebo). There was no difference in death from any cause or stroke between the two groups, but the women on raloxifene had a greater risk of fatal strokes than the women on placebo. The risk of clots in the veins was also increased in women on raloxifene, while the risk of vertebral (spinal) fractures was decreased.

My own personal view of the whole estrogen question is that the protective effect of estrogen on the vascular system is quite age specific. That is, estrogen protects the blood vessels of women during their reproductive years, but probably not for very long afterwards. Mother Nature is no dummy, and just as we wouldn't dream of putting a five-year-old girl on estrogen (among other things it would stop the growth of her long bones) we shouldn't dream of putting a 65-year-old woman on estrogen. By 65 years of age most of us have some plaque in our arteries, and estrogen, by increasing the likelihood of blood clots and causing constriction of diseased arteries is more apt to do harm rather than good.

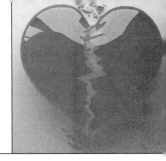

Chapter 6

The Diseased Heart in Greater Depth

In Chapter 2 we discussed atherosclerosis and the build-up of plaque in the arteries. When a coronary artery (an artery that supplies the heart muscle itself) becomes 75% narrowed by plaque, blood flow to the heart becomes insufficient; hence the term "coronary insufficiency" you may have heard bandied about by your doctor. Usually, there's enough blood supply to the heart muscle at rest, but if a person with this degree of plaque starts to exercise, the blood supply to the heart can't increase and that person will begin to experience a symptom that doctors call **angina pectoris** (a Latin term that means a choking or a strangling in the chest). Some people experience this discomfort as a pressure, burning, or heaviness. Some experience no discomfort at all, only shortness of breath. But the hallmark of angina is that it is brought on by exercise or emotional stress, and then goes away within a few minutes with rest, relaxation, or a medicine called nitroglycerin. Women are more likely than men to have angina at rest, during sleep, or in locations other than the chest. We don't know the reason for this.

If your physician suspects that your chest discomfort is angina, she will refer you for testing. The gold standard for diagnosing blockages affecting the coronary arteries is a **cardiac catheterization** and **coronary angiogram**. In this procedure, which is discussed in more detail in Chapter 8, x-ray movie pictures are taken of the coronary arteries to determine if they have plaque build-up that's starving the heart for blood.

This relative lack of blood supply is called ischemia and it can affect any organ system in the body. In simple terms, ischemia means an imbalance between blood supply and demand. Angina is the symptom people usually experience when their hearts are ischemic. A transient ischemic attack (TIA) occurs when there's a brief imbalance between the supply of blood to the brain and what the brain needs. Such an attack can be a warning that a stroke is about to occur. When there is insufficient blood flow to the legs, people commonly experience pain in the calves or buttocks upon walking. This pain is referred to as intermittent claudication, and is a symptom of ischemia, in this case affecting the lower extremities. In the vast majority of cases, ischemia is caused by the build-up of atherosclerotic plaque in the arteries.

In addition to obstruction caused by the build-up of plaque, arteries can be transiently narrowed due to spasm. The smooth muscle in an artery can contract to such a degree that the artery is severely narrowed or in some cases completely blocked. For reasons that we don't understand, this condition is more common in women. Cocaine use has also been shown to cause coronary spasm. Several years ago I treated a young man who snorted cocaine on his wedding night. He developed severe chest pain and was hospitalized with a heart attack. A short time later a coronary angiogram found no evidence of clot or plaque. Since my encounter with this patient, there have been multiple reports in the medical literature of cocaine-induced heart disease.

As we saw in Chapter 2, plaques that develop in the arteries can rupture. When this happens a clot usually forms over the area where plaque material gets exposed to the blood stream. If a large enough clot forms and totally blocks the artery, the tissue supplied by that artery can die, often with catastrophic results. When heart muscle dies from interruption of its blood supply physicians call this a myocardial infarction (MI). (You may be more familiar with the term "heart attack.") If blood flow isn't restored within a few hours, either by clot-dissolving medicines or by angioplasty, the heart muscle dies. Over the next few weeks the heart heals by forming a tough scar, but the scar tissue can't contract like normal heart muscle, so the rest of the heart has to work harder to maintain circulation.

If so much heart muscle is destroyed that the heart can no longer pump sufficient blood for the body's needs, congestive heart failure (CHF) occurs. The most common symptom of CHF is shortness of breath with exertion. The medical term for shortness of breath is **dyspnea**. Dyspnea occurs because when the heart is damaged it becomes stiff. This causes the pressure in the heart to become abnormally elevated, and this pressure is transmitted back into the lungs. Sometimes the pressure becomes so high that fluid oozes out of the lung capillaries into the air sacs, causing extreme shortness of breath and a rattling sound when the affected person breathes. This tends to occur during the night. When a person wakes up gasping for breath, physicians call this **paroxysmal nocturnal dyspnea** (PND). PND is almost always a sign of significant heart failure. The right ventricle may also fail (most often in response to prolonged failure of the left ventricle) and when this occurs the kidneys respond by holding on to salt and water, causing **edema** (swelling).

Angina pectoris is usually the first symptom of coronary artery disease (CAD) in women. In contrast, heart attacks and sudden death are more often the first signs of CAD in men. Women are more apt than men to experience angina in the back or the jaw. When women have heart attacks, they're more likely to have silent heart attacks (heart attacks without any pain) and are more likely than men to have nausea and vomiting or even just severe fatigue as the first symptoms of a heart attack.

There are other important differences between heart disease in men and women. On average, CAD presents in women ten to twenty years later than it does in men. As we've discussed in Chapter 5, women before the age of menopause are less likely than men of the same age to have CAD. However, when young women develop heart attacks, they're more than twice as likely to die from them as men of the same age. Data published by the American Heart Association in 1999 revealed that one third of women age 65 or older had some evidence of CAD. Postmenopausal women are ten times more likely to die of cardiovascular disease than breast cancer.

There are also important differences in cardiovascular health between the races. The death rate from heart disease is 25% to 30% higher for African American women than it is for white women of the same age. The death rate from MI in African American women is twice that of white women.

Although atherosclerosis underlies most cardiac disease in the United States, there are many other conditions that affect the heart. The most common of these is high blood pressure or hypertension, which is more common in men before age 55 but more common in women after age 55. In its sixth report, issued in 1997, the Joint National Committee (JNC)

on Detection, Evaluation, and Treatment of High Blood Pressure, a panel of eminent scientists, defined hypertension as blood pressure greater than 135/85 mm Hg. (The numbers are in millimeters of mercury, the height that a column of mercury will rise to if subjected to the pressure in an artery.) The higher number is the systolic blood pressure, the pressure generated when the heart contracts. (Systole is the term we use to describe that portion of the heart's cycle in which it contracts.) The lower or diastolic pressure is the pressure in the arteries when the heart is relaxed. (Diastole is the term we use to describe that portion of the heart's cycle in which it is relaxed.) An elevation in either number, if untreated over a period of years, is associated with an increased risk of arteriosclerosis, stroke, and kidney failure. In response to the increased work the heart needs to perform in the presence of hypertension, the heart muscle enlarges and thickens. This condition is called left ventricular hypertrophy (LVH) and can be diagnosed by an electrocardiogram (EKG) or other methods. Sometimes the heart muscle becomes so thickened that it outgrows its blood supply. People with this condition can experience angina even in the absence of narrowed arteries. Over time, the thickened ventricle begins to dilate. When this happens, the heart's pump function becomes abnormal and its ability to contract declines. If the person hasn't already succumbed to a stroke or kidney failure, congestive heart failure will ultimately occur. We call the heart disease that results from longstanding hypertension "hypertensive heart disease."

Hypertension becomes more common as we age. Sixty-two percent of white women and 76% of African American women age 65 or older have hypertension, compared to 55% of white men and 65% of African American men at the same age. Most hypertension is what is called "essential," which is a polite way to say that doctors don't have a clue as to what causes it. More than 90% of the hypertension we see falls into this category. This condition tends to run in families but the way it's inherited isn't fully understood.

Obesity also increases the chance of developing hypertension by mechanisms that aren't known. Chronic kidney disease and blockages in the arteries supplying the kidneys can cause hypertension. There are rare tumors of the adrenal gland (a gland that sits near the kidney and produces several hormones) that can cause hypertension. Hypertension may develop during pregnancy, although normally in pregnancy there is a fall in blood pressure. Untreated high blood pressure in pregnancy can cause life-threatening complications for the mother and baby. Lastly, a small percentage of women who take oral contraceptives develop high blood pressure on the pill.

The good news is that there is an array of effective medications that can lower high blood pressure to normal levels. Multiple studies have shown that controlling hypertension lowers mortality and decreases the risk of developing heart attack, stroke, and kidney failure.

Atherosclerotic and hypertensive heart disease are far and away the most common cardiac conditions, but the heart is vulnerable to multiple other diseases and insults. We will discuss some of these less common conditions starting from the outside of the heart and progressing inward.

As described in Chapter 1, the heart is suspended in a thin glistening membrane called the pericardial sac. The tissue that makes up the sac is called the **pericardium**. In rare instances the sac is absent. Sometimes only part of the pericardial sac is missing. This condition can cause an abnormal chest x-ray but rarely causes problems.

The most common condition that affects the pericardium is acute inflammation, called **pericarditis**. The classic signs and symptoms of this disease include chest pain (which is often severe, and is made worse by deep breaths, coughing, or lying down), pericardial rub (a characteristic sound the heart makes that resembles the noise of sand paper on wood), and distinctive abnormalities on the EKG (which may be confused with those that occur with a heart attack).

There are numerous causes of pericarditis. The most common are viral infections, bacterial infections, diseases such as lupus erythematosus (in which the body attacks its own tissue), MI, kidney failure, cancer, an underactive thyroid, and tuberculosis. Pericarditis can also occur after open-heart surgery.

Sometimes the pericardial sac fills up with fluid or pus (or blood, especially in people taking blood thinners) in response to inflammation or infection. If fluid accumulates rapidly, the pericardial sac becomes tense and distended, thus putting pressure on the heart and interfering with its ability to pump. This causes severe shortness of breath and weakness. **Pericardial tamponade** is the term given to this condition. It's an emergency situation that requires the removal of the fluid either by a needle or surgery. If the fluid around the heart accumulates slowly, massive amounts can be present before shortness of breath, weakness, and fatigue occur.

Chronic constrictive pericarditis is an uncommon condition in which the pericardial layers become thickened and stiff, again putting pressure on the heart and limiting its ability to function. People with this disease may experience severe fatigue and marked swelling of the legs and abdomen along with shortness of breath on exertion. They may have an unusual heart sound called a pericardial knock. This condition is insidious and has multiple causes, including all of the conditions that can cause acute pericarditis. It can also occur in people who have had radiation therapy to the chest for cancer. Most of the time, however, the cause is unknown. This condition is treated by surgically removing the diseased pericardium.

The **myocardium** or heart muscle can also be affected by a multitude of diseases other than the most common: ischemic heart disease and hypertensive heart disease. A primary abnormality of the heart muscle is called a **cardiomyopathy**, and there are many possible causes. Again, many are what doctors call **idiopathic** (of unknown origin), an impressive term to cloak our ignorance of their cause. There are also hereditary cardiomyopathies, the genetics of which are currently being studied. There are some cardiomyopathies for which we know the cause. These forms can be treated successfully. Chief among these are the cardiomyopathies caused by alcohol abuse, an underactive thyroid (**hypothyroidism**), and iron overload disease (**hemochromatosis**). All of these types of cardiomyopathies can cause severe congestive heart failure. All three should be looked for in anyone who has what appears to be a cardiomyopathy because all can be treated or cured.

Alcoholic cardiomyopathy is the most common treatable cause of cardiomyopathy in the western world. Complete abstention from alcohol results in recovery in many people who haven't developed severe heart failure. But once people who abuse alcohol develop advanced heart failure, they must quit or die: if they continue to drink, more than three-quarters will be dead within three years. Women who develop alcoholic cardiomyopathy seem to do so at a lower cumulative lifetime dose of alcohol compared with men.

The heart failure caused by an underactive thyroid is completely reversible with thyroid replacement, in which the patient takes supplemental hormones to replace the hormones that the thyroid should be making, but isn't. Cardiomyopathy caused by iron overload is treated by regular bloodletting, one of the few situations where this ancient remedy is truly indicated and helpful.

Viral infections of the heart can cause heart damage. In some cases, the damage is self-limited and ends when the infection is cured; in other cases it's ongoing and is felt to be the cause of some of the so-called idiopathic cardiomyopathy that we see.

There is one cardiomyopathy that affects only women. It's called **peripartum cardiomyopathy** and occurs in the last trimester of pregnancy or within six months of delivery. This condition is thought to be an autoimmune disease, in which the body attacks its own tissues. The body has the ability to recognize foreign tissue. When it does so, it manufactures antibodies, which are proteins that attack and destroy the invaders. This process is called the immune response. People who receive organ transplants need to be on medication to combat this immune response so that their bodies don't reject the tissues of the transplanted organ (unless their transplanted organ comes from an identical twin who is genetically and immunologically indistinguishable). The uterus, like the heart, is made up of many muscles. Sometimes in the latter weeks of pregnancy, proteins from the uterine muscle leak into the mother's bloodstream. Some women manufacture antibodies against these uterine muscle proteins, which are similar to the proteins that make the heart contract. The antibodies then attack heart cells causing the heart muscle to weaken and dilate. Viral infection is also thought to be a cause of this form of cardiomyopathy.

Peripartum cardiomyopathy is treated with bed rest and medications. Luckily, this condition is rare, occurring in between 1/1,300 and 1/15,000 pregnancies. Women over 35, African-American women, those carrying twins or triplets, malnourished women, and women with high blood pressure have a higher risk of developing this disease. In about one half of cases, the heart returns to normal within six months of delivery.

Unfortunately, some women never recover and go on to develop chronic congestive heart failure with a death rate of 85% within five years. Among women whose hearts don't return to normal functioning, future pregnancies are associated with a 50% risk of maternal death. Even in women whose heart function returns to normal, subsequent pregnancy is associated with a 10% risk of death. For these reasons, a woman with peripartum cardiomyopathy is advised to avoid future pregnancies. Cardiac transplantation can be performed in those women who go on to develop severe congestive heart failure. Cardiac transplantation is the treatment of last resort for all eligible patients with end-stage incurable cardiomyopathies (see Chapter 11).

There is another form of cardiomyopathy that occurs much more frequently in women than men. While it has been well known in Japan for a long time, it has only been recognized in this country over the last few years. The Japanese named it **Takotsubo cardiomyopathy** because the appearance of the left ventricle on an angiogram resembles an octopus trap, and takotsubo is the Japanese name for these jar-shaped traps. Most people with this syndrome experience chest pain and dyspnea. They may have slight elevations of the enzymes that leak into the blood in the course of a heart attack, but the degree of heart failure, and the abnormality seen on the left ventricular angiogram is out of proportion to the enzyme leak. Coronary angiograms do not reveal plaque or clots in the coronary arteries. Over the course of days to weeks, the heart function usually improves dramatically. The onset of this condition is often preceded by a sudden emotional trauma or physical stress. Women are affected about nine times more often than men. The average age of patients with Takotsubo cardiomyopathy has ranged from 58 to 77 years. While the cause is unknown, increased levels of the sympathetic hormone norepinephrine have been found in many people suffering from this disorder.

The interior of the heart contains valves that keep the blood flowing in the proper direction. On the left side of the heart are the mitral (named after a bishop's tall hat, or miter, which it was felt to resemble) and aortic valves. On the right side are the tricuspid and pulmonic valves. Two things, neither good, can happen to the valves: they can become leaky (regurgitant) or they can become narrowed (stenotic). Malfunctioning valves cause distinctive sounds, called heart murmurs, which the doctor can hear with the stethoscope. Both leaky and narrowed valves put an extra workload on the heart, which over time can lead to congestive heart failure.

Before the antibiotic age, the most likely cause of damaged valves was a disease called rheumatic fever. Rheumatic fever can develop in certain susceptible children and young adults. Initially the disease starts as a throat infection caused by some strains of strep bacteria (the medical name for this germ is Streptococcus). One to five weeks after an episode of strep throat, fever, arthritis, rash, nodules in the skin, and signs of inflammation of the heart and valves develop. The initial attack of rheumatic fever may be followed by recurrent attacks with subsequent strep infections.

Rheumatic fever is felt to be an autoimmune disease. The antibodies produced to fight the infectious bacteria mistakenly attack cardiac tissue. Years later, people who have had rheumatic fever can develop leaky or narrowed valves. Interestingly, the mitral valve is more commonly affected in women and the aortic valve is more commonly affected in men with rheumatic heart disease.

It's less common for the tricuspid and pulmonic valves to be deformed by rheumatic heart disease. Widespread treatment of sore throats with antibiotics has led to a marked reduction in the incidence of rheumatic fever. Today, it's rare to see a case in the United States. Unfortunately, in much of the developing world rheumatic fever continues to take a devastating toll of lives.

Cardiac valves can also become infected. Infection is especially likely to occur in valves that are deformed for whatever cause and this condition is called infective endocarditis (IE). Doctors used to instruct anyone with a heart murmur due to a deformed valve, even if the degree of deformity was mild, to take antibiotics before any procedure likely to put bacteria into the blood stream, such as dental procedures or surgery on the bowel. However, in October 2007 the American Heart Association published revised guidelines for the prevention of IE. Currently, the only people who need to take prophylactic antiobiotics to prevent IE are those with artificial heart valves, a history of IE, certain forms of congenital heart disease and certain people who have had a cardiac transplantation.

Before the antibiotic era, IE was uniformly fatal. My father's mother died of this disease in 1925, when he was five years old and she was pregnant with her third child. I like to think that she would be delighted to know that her granddaughter has cured several people of the disease that took her life and left her two children orphaned at a tender age.

When IE does occur, we treat it with a prolonged course of antibiotics. The most likely valves to be infected are the mitral and aortic. Intravenous drug abusers, however, have a higher rate of infections involving the valves on the right side of the heart.

Mitral valve prolapse (MVP) is a condition in which the mitral valve balloons back into the left atrium when the left ventricle contracts. It is often diagnosed when the physician hears a clicking sound on listening to the heart. The diagnosis is then confirmed by an **echocardiogram**, a test that uses sound waves to construct a moving image of the heart. MVP is two times more common in women than men.

MVP can be congenital (that is you can be born with it) or it can be acquired. It's the most common form of congenital heart defect. The most common cause of acquired MVP is coronary heart disease. This occurs when the valve's supporting structure is damaged in the course of a heart attack. There are also a host of familial diseases that can make people prone to MVP.

People with mitral valve prolapse are often troubled by symptoms of chest pain and a sensation of fluttering in the chest (what doctors call palpitations). It is usually, but not always, easy to distinguish the chest pain associated with MVP from that associated with angina pectoris. MVP pain is usually sporadic, sharp, and not brought on by exertion.

The palpitations that people with MVP experience are usually caused by extra heartbeats. These extra beats, called **premature contractions,** can arise in the atria or ventricles. People with MVP also appear to have a higher incidence of panic attacks. In rare instances, small clots can form in the folds of a prolapsed mitral valve. These clots may break off and travel to the brain, causing strokes. Any stroke-like symptom in a young person should prompt a search for MVP. There are various medications that can be used when patients with MVP are troubled by palpitations. These drugs are discussed in Chapter 9. In rare instances, the prolapsing mitral valve becomes extremely leaky and needs to be surgically repaired or replaced.

With the aging of the population, another heart valve abnormality has become increasingly common: calcific aortic stenosis. This narrowing of the aortic valve causes progressive obstruction of blood flow from the left ventricle. It is now the most common valve abnormality requiring valve replacement. In calcific aortic stenosis, calcium deposits build up in the aortic valve over time, causing it to become obstructed. Men are about two times more likely to have calcific aortic stenosis than women.

In order for blood to move past the narrowed valve, the heart has to beat more vigorously. The blood is pushed through the narrowed opening and this causes a characteristic murmur that your physician can hear.

Surgical replacement of the valve prolongs life and improves symptoms. The most common symptoms of calcific aortic stenosis are angina, shortness of breath upon exercise, and fainting. These occur late in the course of the disease and are always an indication that the valve needs to be replaced. Your physician can gain a lot of information about the state of the heart and its valves with an echocardiogram (a diagnostic test that uses sound waves to construct an image of the heart; see Chapter 8) but when aortic valve replacement is being considered in anyone middle aged or older, a cardiac catheterization should also be performed to determine if any coronary arteries are blocked.

The aortic valve can also be leaky. (In fact valves can be both narrowed and leaky.) Two terms you may hear to describe a leaking valve are regurgitation and insufficiency. There are many conditions that can cause the aortic valve to leak. Before the invention of antibiotics, rheumatic fever and syphilis were two of the most common causes. Infection of the aortic valve can cause acute severe aortic insufficiency. Some people are born with aortic valves that are abnormal. The most common congenital abnormality of the aortic valve is a "bicuspid aortic valve." In this condition, which is more common in males, there are only two aortic valve leaflets (cusps) rather than the normal three. These abnormal bicuspid valves can become both narrowed and/or leaky, usually in middle age. The most common cause of aortic regurgitation nowadays is disease that affects the root of the aorta (the part of the aorta that arises just above the aortic valve). Certain medical conditions can cause the aortic root to dilate. The most common of these is hypertension. Marked dilatation of the aortic root causes the three leaflets of the aortic valve to separate, thus allowing blood to leak back into the left ventricle when the heart is resting between beats. This puts increased strain on the heart, causing it to enlarge and eventually fail.

A few years ago, two medications prescribed to suppress appetite in overweight people were discovered to have a terrible, unforeseen side effect: they sometimes caused the cardiac valves to become leaky. These drugs, fenfluramine and dexfenfluramine (marketed under the names Pondimin and Redux) were taken by millions of people, mostly women. Fenfluramine was also prescribed with another medication, phentermine, a combination that was popularly known as "fen-phen." The Centers for Disease Control and Prevention issued an alert in 1997 after more than one hundred cases of leaky valves were reported in people taking either fenfluramine or dexfenfluramine. Of those who reported problems, 86% had aortic regurgitation; 19% had **mitral regurgitation** either alone or in combination with aortic regurgitation. Out of the total cases reported, 98% of leaky valves were found in women; 24% of those affected required cardiac valve replacement surgery. These drugs were eventually taken off the market, but not before some people died.

The symptoms of aortic regurgitation are similar to those of aortic stenosis, but fainting is less common. A leaky aortic valve causes a characteristic murmur, which usually alerts the physician to the presence of the condition. People may not experience symptoms until very late in the disease, so regular follow-up is important. Surgery is most successful if it's performed before the heart has begun to fail.

The mitral valve, which directs the flow of blood from the left atrium to the left ventricle, can also become narrowed, leaky, or both. When the valve is narrowed the condition is called **mitral stenosis.** Ninety-nine percent of narrowed mitral valves are caused by rheumatic heart disease, and two thirds of patients with rheumatic mitral stenosis (MS) are women. MS can also be congenital, but this is diagnosed in infants and young children. Very rarely, MS is caused by an unusual tumor called malignant carcinoid; it can also occur as a complication of autoimmune diseases like lupus erythematosus and in certain familial diseases. Symptoms occur earlier in the course of mitral stenosis than in aortic valve disease. The principal symptom of MS is shortness of breath on exertion. This dyspnea may be associated with a cough or wheezing, and sometimes with the coughing up of blood. People with MS may have shortness of breath when they lie down (**orthopnea**) and may be awakened with attacks of severe **paroxysmal nocturnal dyspnea**. They are prone to develop an abnormally rapid heartbeat, a specific abnormal rhythm called **atrial fibrillation**. Atrial fibrillation, along with other stresses such as infection, pregnancy, fever, or exercise can cause people with MS to develop life threatening heart failure. Medicine to lower the heart rate can enable some people with MS to become symptom free and to postpone surgery.

The left atrium becomes progressively enlarged as mitral stenosis worsens. The pressure in the left atrium rises and this pressure is transmitted back to the lungs, causing shortness of breath. The enlargement of the left atrium predisposes to the development of atrial fibrillation. Clots may form in this situation, and if they break off and travel to the brain they can cause a stroke.

A clot that travels from its site of origin is called an embolus and the process is called **embolization**. The tendency to **embolization** increases with age, with increasing size of the left atrium, and with increasing severity of heart failure. About 80% of the people with MS who develop emboli are in atrial fibrillation. Embolism may occur in people with only mild degrees of stenosis and may be the first symptom of MS. In addition to traveling to the brain, clots may lodge in the coronary arteries, or the arteries supplying other organs such as the kidneys or spleen. People with MS and atrial fibrillation should be treated with a blood thinner called warfarin (Coumadin) which has been proven to lower the risk of embolism.

In temperate climates, symptoms of rheumatic MS develop approximately 15 to 20 years after the acute attack of rheumatic fever. It then usually takes another 5 to 10 years for symptoms to become severe. In the tropics and subtropics, the progression from rheumatic fever to symptoms is much more rapid. Severe mitral stenosis has been diagnosed in children as young as 6 in India. Climate is not the only factor because rapid progression has also been found among the Alaskan Inuit people. But in the United States people usually develop symptoms of MS when they are between the ages of 45 and 65.

Echocardiograms can be used to follow the progression of mitral stenosis. When the valve becomes critically narrowed either surgical replacement or a procedure called **valvulotomy** is indicated. This mechanical opening of the narrowed valve can be performed with a special balloon catheter or surgically.

Mitral regurgitation can occur in rheumatic heart disease; it is more apt to occur in men than women in this setting, unlike MS. Today, however, mitral regurgitation is much more likely to occur due to other causes.

Many conditions predispose a person to the development of a leaky mitral valve. Whenever the left ventricle dilates, the mitral valve can no longer close properly, resulting in mitral regurgitation. Infection, heart attacks, connective tissue disorders, degenerative disorders, and even trauma may all cause mitral regurgitation. If MR occurs abruptly, as in a heart attack, it can be fatal. More often, MR develops slowly, and the heart may be well compensated for years. Fatigue and chronic weakness are more prominent than shortness of breath in people with chronic mitral regurgitation. Patients with mitral regurgitation need to have careful follow-up with regular echocardiograms so that the valve can be repaired or replaced before irreversible heart damage occurs.

Tricuspid regurgitation occurs when the tricuspid valve becomes leaky. This usually happens in response to failure and enlargement of the right ventricle. Failure of the right ventricle can result from severe lung disease, longstanding failure of the left ventricle, or a pulmonary embolism (when a clot travels to the lungs). Intravenous drug abusers are prone to infections on the tricuspid valve from the use of non-sterile needles, and these infections often cause the tricuspid valve to become leaky. Tricuspid valve narrowing or stenosis can also occur, but is much less common than mitral stenosis. Chronic weakness and fatigue occur with tricuspid stenosis or insufficiency. A leaky tricuspid valve causes the liver to pulsate and enlarge, causing swelling of the abdomen and legs. In severe cases, the tricuspid valve can be repaired or replaced surgically.

Primary tumors that originate in the heart are rare. They're found in about 0.002% to 0.3% of autopsies. It's more common for tumors to spread to the heart from some other site, that is, to **metastasize**. Autopsy series show the heart to be involved by metastases in anywhere from 1% to 20% of people with cancer. However, autopsies demonstrate cardiac involvement in up to 60% of people with malignant melanoma, the deadliest form of skin cancer. Other cancers that can spread to the heart, either through the blood or by direct extension, include lung, breast, leukemia, and lymphoma.

The most common type of primary heart tumor is the **myxoma**. Myxomas are usually benign, which means that they will not spread to other parts of the body as cancerous tumors will, but because of their location they can cause life-threatening problems. Almost 90% of myxomas occur in the left atrium, but they may occur elsewhere in the heart. Myxomas can interfere with the mitral and tricuspid valves, causing obstruction to flow or regurgitation. The symptoms can mimic those seen in other heart diseases, but myxomas also cause nonspecific signs and symptoms such as fever, weight loss, pain in the joints, fatigue, and rash. It's not unusual for tumor fragments to break off and travel to the brain and elsewhere. Sometimes, a stroke is the first sign of the tumor. Particularly in a young person with no risk factors, a stroke should raise the question of myxoma.

Most people with myxomas are female (70%), and the average age of diagnosis is around age 55. The cause is unknown, but there are familial cases of myxoma, which make up about 10% of the total.

The diagnosis of cardiac myxoma is usually made by an echocardiogram, which was often ordered for other reasons. The case I remember best was a young woman who had chest pain and palpitations. She had visited emergency departments with these complaints on many occasions and had been assured that her symptoms were due to anxiety. Finally, her physician ordered an echocardiogram thinking that she might have MVP. The echocardiogram showed a large left atrial myxoma that had caused severe damage to her mitral valve. She had emergency surgery to remove the tumor and replace the mitral valve the very next day.

Because myxomas may be familial, if you are diagnosed with a myxoma, all of your family members should have echocardiograms to be certain they aren't affected. The only treatment is surgical excision of the tumor.

A congenital heart defect is one with which you're born. Before the advent of cardiac surgery in the 1960s, most congenital heart disease wasn't curable. Children with severe congenital defects often did not survive to adulthood. Today, more and more congenital heart defects can be corrected surgically, so these babies are surviving and, in the case of females, often having children themselves. At present, about 85% of infants with congenital heart disease will reach adulthood. The number of adults with congenital heart defects is increasing by 5% per year. Excluding cases of MVP, in the year 2000 there were approximately 900,000 adults with congenital heart disease in the United States.

The most likely congenital heart defect to escape detection in childhood is an **atrial septal defect (ASD)**, which is a hole in the wall separating the left and right atria. This abnormality is three times more common in females than males. Unless the defect is very large, infants and children with the defect often have no symptoms. By young adulthood, women with ASDs develop fatigue, although pregnancy is usually well tolerated. By about age 40, many people with an ASD develop abnormal heart rhythms; unless the defect is corrected, their health usually goes downhill and they develop heart failure. If the defect is not corrected, the average age at death is 55 for the most common type of ASD.

Of those with an ASD, 20% to 60% will also have MVP. One dreaded complication of an ASD is a so-called paradoxical embolism. In the absence of an opening between the atria, if a clot in a vein, for example in the legs, breaks off and travels to the heart, it will lodge in the lungs, a **pulmonary embolus**. This is obviously not a good thing, but if the clot is not large, the lungs can recover. However, with an opening between the atria, a clot arising from the venous system can now travel to the left side of the heart and wind up in the brain, causing a stroke. This is another situation in which a stroke in a young person should prompt the doctor to order an echocardiogram, which is a safe and accurate way to diagnose an ASD or a more common condition called a patent foramen ovale (PFO). The foramen ovale is an opening in the septum or wall between the atria, which in fetal life allows oxygenated blood from the placenta to cross over to the left side of the heart, from whence it is pumped around the body. Normally, the foramen ovale closes at birth or soon after, but in some people a small opening remains. Just as with an ASD, clots originating in a vein can gain access to the arterial system through a PFO and cause a stroke.

Surgery, or nowadays more frequently catheter based therapies, can close ASDs and PFOs. Closure of the defect allows for a normal life span.

A ventricular septal defect (VSD) occurs when a hole develops between the ventricles. This condition is usually diagnosed in infancy and is well tolerated if the defect is small. In fact, many small defects close spontaneously. Large holes, however, need to be closed surgically because high pressure may develop in the lung arteries, a process that can cause irreversible damage. A woman with a small VSD can usually go through pregnancy without problem.

Coarctation of the aorta is another relatively common congenital defect. This is a narrowing in the aorta as it travels through the chest. It causes high blood pressure and a difference in the blood pressure measured in the arms versus the legs. (Blood pressure in the legs should be similar to that in the arms.) Most cases are diagnosed in childhood. Males with this condition outnumber females by two to one.

The optimal age for repair is between 3 and 5 years. Between 30% and 60% of patients with coarctation of the aorta also have a deformed, bicuspid aortic valve. People with coarctation of the aorta die at an average age of 35 if it isn't repaired. Among untreated people with this condition over the age of 40, 90% have high blood pressure and almost 70% have congestive heart failure. Surgical correction should be performed even in older people. People with a history of coarctation of the aorta should have echocardiograms to look for a deformed aortic valve. If one is found, they should be closely observed for the development of aortic stenosis or insufficiency.

There is another condition of the aorta that is more common in men than women, but has an unexplained propensity to affect pregnant women. The condition is called aortic dissection; it consists of a tear in the inner lining of the aorta, which allows blood to travel between the layers and sometimes to rupture through the aortic wall, causing death rapidly if untreated. It occurs with greater frequency in people with inherited disorders of connective tissue (the tissues that bind cells to each other). The most common of these is called Marfan's Syndrome, which occurs in about 1 in 10,000 live births in the U.S. People with this disorder are frequently tall with long extremities and fingers, and 60% to 80% of women with Marfan's Syndrome have mitral valve prolapse (MVP). Women with Marfan's Syndrome are at high risk of aortic dissection during the latter stages of pregnancy or in the first months after delivery. About half of all aortic dissections in women under the age of 40 occur in association with pregnancy. High blood pressure, coarctation of the aorta, and a bicuspid aortic valve also predispose to aortic dissection. The most common symptom is severe chest pain, occurring suddenly, often described as "tearing" and often radiating to the back. Most aortic dissections can be diagnosed by echocardiography or a special type of x-ray called a CT angiogram (see Chapter 8). They are usually fatal if not operated upon.

Primary Pulmonary Hypertension (PPH) is a disease of unknown cause that occurs more often in women than men. Young women, between the ages of 10 and 40, are most often affected. It is a rare progressive condition in which the pressure in the pulmonary arteries is elevated, eventually causing the right ventricle to fail.

Usually, when the pressure in the pulmonary arteries is increased above normal this is caused by abnormalities on the left side of the heart, such as mitral valve disease, or disease in the lungs, such as emphysema. But in PPH the left side of the heart is normal and there is no disease of the lung tissue to account for the increased pressure in the pulmonary arteries. There are cases of PPH that are genetically linked, and the gene responsible for familial PPH has been identified, but most cases occur sporadically. The diet drugs aminorex in Europe, and fenfluramines in the United States were implicated in outbreaks of PPH in some people who took those drugs and they were taken off the market. Large pulmonary emboli can cause acute pulmonary hypertension, and chronic small pulmonary emboli can mimic PPH.

The earliest symptom of PPH is usually shortness of breath. People with this condition may also experience fatigue, fainting, cough, chest pain, and swelling of the legs or abdomen. The diagnosis of PPH may be suspected by the symptoms and findings on an echocardiogram and EKG, but definitive diagnosis usually involves a cardiac catheterization with measurement of the pressures on the right side of the heart. In addition, the response of the pulmonary artery pressure to medication can be determined during a catheterization, allowing doctors to choose which medicines are most effective.

In the past, PPH was usually rapidly progressive, with death occurring within a few years of diagnosis. During the 1990's newer, more effective drugs to treat PPH became available and nowadays the outlook for people with PPH is much improved. These new medicines for PPH will be discussed in Chapter 9.

Arrhythmias (abnormal heart rhythms) occur in all age groups but increase in frequency with increasing age. Arrhythmias can be further classified as **tachycardias** (the heart beats abnormally fast) or **bradycardias** (the heart beats abnormally slow). In either case, if you develop an abnormal heart rhythm, you may experience a fluttering sensation in the chest. If the heart is beating so fast or so slow that it can't pump sufficient blood to the brain, you lose consciousness. If blood flow to the brain ceases for more than about four minutes, you die. Fortunately, most arrhythmias do not cause death, but they may make you uncomfortable, frightened, or weak to the point of passing out. Passing out should always prompt an evaluation to see if an abnormal heart rhythm is the cause.

A common cause of sudden cardiac death is an arrhythmia called ventricular fibrillation (VF). It usually occurs in the setting of ischemia (remember that word means a relative lack of blood supply) or acute myocardial infarction. There are certain familial disorders that are associated with a propensity for sudden death due to VF. The best studied of these is called "Long QT Syndrome." Several well-publicized deaths of athletes have been attributed to VF associated with cardiomyopathy or drug (cocaine) abuse. Blunt trauma to the chest, which occurs sometimes in sports, can also cause a fatal episode of VF if the trauma happens during a particular part of the cardiac cycle.

The treatment of arrhythmias has been revolutionized by the introduction of pacemakers and implantable devices that can shock the heart back into a normal rhythm. These devices are discussed in Chapter 11.

Now that you have a brief overview of cardiac diseases, you can learn about the signs and symptoms of heart disease. Chapter 7 will help you determine if the symptom you are experiencing is coming from your heart or has a more benign explanation. Obviously, you need to discuss any unusual symptoms with your physician, but in the next chapter you'll learn which symptoms to take seriously and which you may choose to tolerate or ignore.

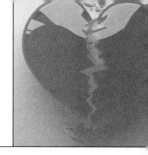

Chapter 7

Signs and Symptoms of Heart Disease: The Chest Pain Conundrum

One definition of the word conundrum is "an intricate and difficult problem." This is what chest pain has proven to be for women. Data from the Framingham Study and other epidemiologic studies seemed to show that angina pectoris was a much less serious problem in women than men. Women who had chest pain in these studies were less likely to develop a heart attack or to die from cardiac disease than men. Other studies that looked at the results of cardiac catheterizations showed that women with chest pain were far more likely than men to have what appeared to be normal coronary arteries. In the Coronary Artery Surgery Study, 50% of women who were referred for coronary angiography for chest pain had little or no evidence of coronary atherosclerosis compared to 17% of men. These data were confirmed by other studies that found coronary angiography for chest pain was more likely to reveal normal arteries in women than in men. This contributed to a false sense of security in women and their

Women and their physicians have had a false sense of security when it comes to chest pain.

physicians when it came to the complaint of chest pain. Because of such studies, women and their physicians were less likely to believe that chest pain was being caused by heart disease.

The original population in the Framingham Study didn't include any women older than age 62. Early reports from the Framingham Study found that in general, women with angina in the Framingham population fared better than men. However, when sufficient time had elapsed so that more older women were included, it became apparent that women older than 65 with angina pectoris had the same poor prognosis as did men. The apparent benign outlook for angina pectoris only applied to younger women.

So, what might be going on in women who have chest pain but no blockages on coronary angiography? In the past, such women were commonly labeled "anxious" or "hysteric" or were said to have "non-cardiac" chest pain. Recent studies, however, have shown that as many as 50% of these women may be suffering from what is called "microvascular dysfunction," a disorder in smaller coronary blood vessels that can lead to debilitating symptoms. Despite the absence of obstructions in the larger coronary arteries on an angiogram, many of these women have objective evidence of ischemia. Their pain is real cardiac pain. Some of these women have had a special kind of test called an *intravascular ultrasound (IVUS)* of their coronary arteries in the course of a cardiac catheterization. Sometimes, despite the absence of severe obstruction the IVUS reveals a great deal of plaque in the artery. This is thought to prevent the artery from dilating appropriately in response to an increased need for blood flow. So even though their arteries may look as if they are not severely narrowed, these women may still suffer from ischemia.

We also know that women are more likely than men to have angina caused by spasm of a coronary artery. The absence of coronary blockages doesn't mean that the angina isn't cardiac in origin. Today, doctors and patients are becoming more aware of the seriousness of chest pain in women.

Although the incidence of coronary artery disease (CAD) is low in women before menopause, it is not zero; every complaint of chest pain must be investigated. This is particularly true for any woman who has risk factors for cardiovascular disease (CVD). Unfortunately, because the high risk of CAD in postmenopausal women wasn't appreciated until fairly recently, many older women were denied appropriate evaluation with coronary angiography. At the same time, a number of younger women with no risk factors for CAD were subjected to angiograms when there was little chance that they had significant obstructions in their coronary arteries.

There are certain characteristics that can help you determine if your chest discomfort could be coming from your heart. The hallmark of angina pectoris is that usually it's precipitated by exertion or stress and promptly (within five minutes) relieved by rest. In addition, angina tends NOT to be felt as a sharp pain. It's more commonly perceived as a tightness, heaviness, or squeezing discomfort. Anginal pain doesn't increase with coughing or deep breaths, although it may be worse lying down than sitting up or standing. Angina pectoris is usually accompanied by a feeling of shortness of breath. As for location, angina pectoris can be felt anywhere in the upper body. When it starts in the chest it can radiate into the arms, neck, or jaw. Women with angina pectoris are more likely than men to have jaw, neck, or back discomfort, without any chest discomfort. I have had patients complain of pain in the wrists or in the upper abdomen; their symptoms turned out to be angina.

If discomfort isn't brought on or worsened by physical exercise or stress, isn't associated with shortness of breath, isn't located above the waist, and isn't of relatively short duration (5 or 10 minutes), it is unlikely to be angina. However, women with CAD are more likely than men to experience angina pectoris with emotional stress, at rest, or awakening them from sleep.

Pay close attention to the characteristics of any chest pain you experience. The more accurately you can describe what you're feeling, the more likely it will be that your doctor will arrive at the correct diagnosis. Don't be satisfied with a diagnosis of anxiety if your discomfort has the characteristics of angina pectoris, particularly if you're postmenopausal or premenopausal with multiple risk factors. Insist on being evaluated for the possibility of heart disease. Nothing is gained when you or your physician minimize the seriousness of chest pain.

The more accurately you can describe what you're feeling, the more likely it will be that your doctor will arrive at the correct diagnosis.

Don't forget that there are conditions other than CAD that can cause chest pain. Common ones include mitral valve prolapse (MVP) and acid reflux into the esophagus, among others. Less common conditions may also occur and can be missed if your physician doesn't order the appropriate tests. One of my patients had multiple visits to area emergency departments and her primary care physician for chest pain before an echocardiogram was ordered. It revealed a tumor of the heart that would have been fatal if she hadn't undergone surgery.

Unlike angina pectoris, the pain associated with a myocardial infarction (MI)—also known as a heart attack—is commonly severe and prolonged. The pain of an MI may be associated with profuse sweating and a feeling of impending doom. Women are less likely than men to report sweating as a symptom associated with heart attack, but are more likely to have nausea, palpitations, and jaw, neck, or back pain. Unfortunately, about 30% of heart attacks in women go unrecognized at the time. Some of these are so-called "silent" MIs, which occur without pain. The Framingham Study found that 34% of women's MIs were unrecognized, compared with 27% of men's. In addition, silent MIs increased the risk for complications such as stroke, heart failure, or death.

An interesting article was published in the journal *Circulation* in 2003. Investigators surveyed 515 women 4 to 6 months after MI. The authors reported that only 28% of these women had the classic substernal (under the breast bone) chest pain. In fact, the most common symptom was shortness of breath which was reported as the main symptom by 58% of women. In addition, almost 80% of these women had symptoms for a month or more prior to their MI and the most common of these was unusual fatigue, occurring in 71%.

Severe chest pain is a medical emergency. When in doubt, err on the side of safety and call 911. It's far better to spend a few hours in the emergency department and find out that you're just having a gall bladder attack than to stay home and die of an MI.

Severe chest pain is a medical emergency. When in doubt, err on the side of safety and call 911.

Severe chest pain that worsens with deep breathing (what physicians call pleuritic pain) may be a sign of pericarditis (inflammation of the heart's lining). Pleuritic chest pain can also be the first symptom of a pulmonary embolus (a clot in the lung). In addition, pleuritic chest pain can occur when the pleura, the lining of the lungs, is inflamed, for example from pneumonia. Severe chest pain radiating to the back may be caused by an MI, but it's also felt when the aorta dissects (tears).

Pain isn't the only symptom that can be a clue to the presence of disease. Some people with cardiac disease never experience pain over the entire course of their illness. The next section examines other common symptoms of heart disease as well as some of the signs physicians look for when they examine you. If your physician isn't doing a careful physical examination when you go for a check-up, he or she may be missing important clues to the presence of heart disease.

Medical textbooks define dyspnea as an abnormally uncomfortable awareness of breathing. To simplify, dyspnea is an abnormal shortness of breath. In most cases, dyspnea is a manifestation of either heart or lung disease. At some point in the course of their illness, most people with heart disease experience shortness of breath. For some people, dyspnea is the only symptom that their heart is starved for oxygen. In such circumstances, the person's dyspnea is said to be an anginal equivalent. This is especially common in diabetics, who also have a higher incidence of silent heart attacks than nondiabetics.

Dyspnea can occur suddenly or it can come on so gradually that the person is unaware of any limitation until their disease is far advanced. Sudden dyspnea can be a sign of a pulmonary embolus, heart attack, acute failure of one of the heart's valves, or acute congestive heart failure. People with rheumatic heart disease, in whom the cardiac valves become gradually narrowed or leaky over many years, often have an insidious onset of dyspnea. They slowly cut back on their physical activity and the true extent of their limitation may not be apparent until they undergo formal exercise stress testing. The gradual onset of shortness of breath can also occur with cardiomyopathy. A physician I knew became aware that it was taking him longer than usual to bicycle 25 miles, which he did several times a week, and that the reason was that he was becoming short of breath. This was the first indication of a cardiomyopathy that ultimately proved fatal.

When heart failure is present, people commonly experience orthopnea, shortness of breath that's worse when lying down, and paroxysmal nocturnal dyspnea (PND), the sudden onset of shortness of breath during sleep. PND is also called cardiac asthma. The presence of PND or dyspnea at rest is always a cause for concern. Unfortunately, I can't count the number of women who have consulted me for shortness of breath after being diagnosed with asthma. Even when they didn't improve with asthma medication their physicians didn't think that they might be short of breath from heart disease. One physician told his patient when she complained of shortness of breath: "You're over 70. What do you expect?" Not satisfied with this response, the woman came to me for a second opinion. I ordered a stress test for her, which was very abnormal. She had an angioplasty to open up a narrowed coronary artery. After the procedure, her "asthma" disappeared.

Anyone can experience dyspnea with enough exertion. What you should be on the lookout for is a change in your exercise tolerance. If you could climb four flights of stairs with no problem a year ago, but now are huffing and puffing after two, you have cause for concern. On the other hand, if you can run for an hour without shortness of breath, you can be certain that your heart and lungs are in fine condition.

The *Taber's Medical Dictionary* that my parents gave me when I entered medical school in 1964 defines palpitation as "rapid, violent or throbbing pulsation, as an abnormally rapid throbbing or fluttering of the heart." Some people go through life and are never aware of their heart beating. Others are exquisitely attuned to every hiccup in their heart's rhythm. (These patients generate lots of extra income for cardiologists who, correctly, order 24-hour monitoring of the EKG to be certain that a dangerous abnormal rhythm isn't occurring.)

Most palpitations are caused by extra heartbeats arising either in the atria or the ventricles. These extra beats usually occur earlier than the next normal heartbeat would, so they are called premature contractions. Premature contractions are usually followed by a pause, and the beat following this longer than usual pause is especially forceful (because the heart has had more time to fill up with blood). This especially forceful heart contraction is what causes the throbbing or fluttering sensation, which can be disturbing for the person who experiences it. A good rule of thumb is that if your palpitations are brief, infrequent, and not associated with shortness of breath, dizziness, or fainting, it's likely that the palpitations aren't serious. In the absence of diagnosed heart disease, premature contractions don't carry an ominous prognosis. However, if palpitations are prolonged, occur many times a day, or have associated symptoms as mentioned above, they should be investigated.

The medical term for fainting is **syncope** (pronounced SING-co-pee). True syncope implies loss of consciousness with inability to maintain a standing position. It most commonly occurs when the blood supply to the brain is reduced.

A marked drop in blood pressure or a serious arrhythmia is the usual cause of syncope. However, very low blood glucose and hyperventilation (over breathing) can also cause fainting. Epileptics lose consciousness during an attack, but in that situation typical seizure movements of the arms and legs are usually present. Certain medications used to treat hypertension can cause fainting by lowering the blood pressure too much, especially when someone taking such a medication gets up too quickly from a lying or sitting position. This positional drop in blood pressure is called **orthostatic hypotension.** This condition can also occur in those who are severely dehydrated and in those who have lost a significant amount of blood. When fainting is caused by blockages in the arteries supplying the brain, there are usually other symptoms such as a history of blindness in one eye, or weakness and/or tingling on one side of the body. Fainting can be a symptom of a critically narrowed aortic valve or of abnormally thickened heart muscle. The new onset of fainting in an adult should always trigger a search for the cause.

Perhaps the most common form of fainting is **vasovagal syncope,** which usually occurs in the setting of acute emotional stress. It makes up about one-half of all cases of syncope. This common faint is caused by an imbalance in what's called the autonomic nervous system. This body system controls many important functions, but it isn't under our conscious control. For example, the autonomic nervous system is involved in the "fight or flight" reflex, which helps us respond to sudden threats in our environment. The autonomic nervous system can be further divided into two subsystems: the **sympathetic nervous system** and the **parasympathetic nervous system.** The sympathetic nervous system is activated in situations of danger or stress. The parasympathetic system causes inhibition or slowing of most of the body's processes. In the common faint, the parasympathetic system activates and the sympathetic system is inhibited. The vagus nerve is the main carrier of parasympathetic impulses. When the vagus nerve is activated during vasovagal syncope, the blood vessels dilate causing blood pressure to drop. The heart rate slows and the circulation to the brain is insufficient to maintain consciousness.

Vasovagal syncope rarely occurs when a person is lying down. The sufferer is usually standing or sitting and begins to experience unpleasant sensations such as nausea, blurred vision, weakness, and lightheadedness before blacking out. He or she appears pale and sweaty. Consciousness usually returns promptly when the affected individual lies down, especially if the legs are then elevated. (This maneuver allows the heart to pump more blood.) People with vasovagal syncope usually have a history of episodes dating back many years. It's usually benign and requires no therapy other than avoidance of situations that are likely to provoke it.

In some people, activities such as coughing, urinating, swallowing, and defecating are associated with fainting episodes. The first two tend to occur in men who have chronic lung disease or enlarged prostates. The last two occur in men and women. Various tests may be necessary to determine the cause of syncope. No matter what, fainting is a symptom that should always be reported to your physician.

Lay people tend to think of cough as indicating a problem with the lungs, but in fact cough is frequently a symptom of cardiac disease. When the left ventricle fails or when the mitral valve becomes narrowed, pressure builds up in the tiniest lung blood vessels, called pulmonary capillaries. This increased pressure causes a cough that tends to be dry and is frequently more troublesome at night than during the day. If the left atrium becomes markedly enlarged—as it does in mitral valve disorders—it can press on the pulmonary artery and compress a nerve that travels under it to get to the larynx (the voice box). This pressure on the nerve causes cough and hoarseness.

People with severe acute heart failure typically have a cough that produces pink frothy phlegm, and they experience marked shortness of breath. They literally have to "gasp for breath" and feel that they'll die if their breathing doesn't improve. They're right. This is a medical emergency and you must call 911 and get to the hospital if you have these symptoms.

When the aorta dilates and forms an aortic aneurysm, the aneurysm can compress the air tubes (bronchi), causing a dry cough. When a clot travels to the lung and causes damage, a cough and blood streaked sputum commonly result.

The coughing up of blood is called **hemoptysis**. It may indicate disease of the heart or lungs. It occurs in people with mitral stenosis, sometimes in association with exertion or pregnancy. Massive, life-threatening or fatal hemoptysis can be seen in people who have aortic aneurysms that rupture into the lung. Finally, people on blood thinners or certain drugs that suppress the immune system are more prone to bleeding. Any condition likely to cause cough in such people increases the likelihood of hemoptysis.

Edema occurs when the body retains an excessive amount of fluid in the tissues. It can be found anywhere in the body. The location of edema is helpful in determining its cause. Edema occurs in the setting of congestive heart failure through a series of complex mechanisms involving the heart, the kidneys, the sympathetic nervous system, and the endocrine system. When edema affects the ankles and legs and worsens in the evening, the cause is either heart failure or problems with the veins of the legs. If the heart failure isn't treated or if it worsens, the swelling ascends to involve the thighs, genitals, and eventually the abdomen. In people confined to bed, edema tends to accumulate in the lower back, buttocks, and thighs. Edema that affects only one extremity (either the arm or the leg) is usually due to blockage in a vein or lymph channel.

Generalized edema can occur in kidney, liver, or heart failure. The medical term for generalized edema is anasarca. (Your great-grandparents probably called this condition dropsy.) Weight gain usually precedes the appearance of edema. If you gain two or more pounds in 24 hours, the chances are good that this is fluid retention. I once saw a patient with severe heart failure caused by an underactive thyroid gland. When she was treated with thyroid hormone, she lost 80 pounds of fluid!

Cyanosis (bluish discoloration of the skin) occurs when hemoglobin, the oxygen carrying protein in red blood cells, is abnormal or contains less than normal amounts of oxygen. Cyanosis doesn't always indicate a serious problem. Everyone has had the experience of staying too long in the water on a hot summer day and coming out with blue lips and extremities. In such a situation, exposure to cold air causes the smallest skin arteries to constrict, slowing blood flow and allowing more oxygen to be extracted from the blood. However, cyanosis can also be a sign of significant cardiac or pulmonary disease. Certain congenital heart diseases in which there is shunting (abnormal passage) of blood from the right side of the heart to the left side cause cyanosis. Cyanosis also occurs in the setting of acute congestive heart failure and in many conditions in which lung function is impaired. Less commonly, cyanosis can be due to acquired or inherited abnormalities of hemoglobin. Cyanosis is usually easy to detect, but is less apparent in dark-skinned persons, in which case it may be seen more easily in the tongue or the inside of the eyelid.

In this chapter we have reviewed the most common signs and symptoms of cardiac disease. This knowledge won't make you an astute diagnostician, but it will alert you to the clues that indicate when a serious problem might exist or reassure you that your symptom isn't cause for alarm. When in doubt, discuss your concerns with your physician. Your physician will appreciate your trust in his or her judgment and will order the necessary testing to set both your minds at rest.

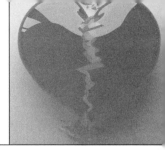

Chapter 8

Diagnostic Tests for Heart Disease: Are There Differences Between Men and Women?

Before we get into a discussion of the most common tests for heart disease, it's important to understand a bit about how such tests are interpreted. To do so, I'm going to give a brief overview of a subject that made my eyes glaze over in medical school, but which nonetheless is vital: statistics. Statistics is a branch of mathematics that deals with the collection and analysis of data. (Mark Twain popularized a saying of England's prime minister at the time. "There are three kinds of lies: lies, damn lies, and statistics.")

When your doctor investigates your symptoms, she orders various tests and interprets the results using her knowledge of statistics. She will have absorbed vast amounts of information from her study of various diseases. She will know that no test is perfect and that the accuracy of any test depends on a number of factors. She will need to know the test's **sensitivity** and **specificity** as well as its predictive value.

When a test is abnormal, we doctors perversely call it a positive test, even though the implication for you is negative. Conversely, when a test is normal, we call it a negative test, even though the implication for you is positive. We say a test is a true positive if the results are abnormal in a person who really does have the disease for which he or she was tested. We say a test is a false positive if the results are abnormal in a person without the disease. A true negative is a test that's normal in someone without the disease. A false negative is a test that's normal in someone with the disease. (Phew! I promise this won't go on much longer.)

Let's use exercise stress tests as an example. Your doctor may order an exercise stress test if it's suspected that you have a blocked coronary artery. The sensitivity of a test refers to the likelihood of the test being abnormal (positive) for the disease being tested. If exercise stress tests were performed on a thousand people with coronary artery disease (CAD), and 900 of them had abnormal test results, the sensitivity of exercise stress testing would be 90%. This means that the test is sensitive enough to pick up CAD in 90% of those who have it. The **sensitivity** of a test is defined as the ratio of true positives to the sum of the true positives and false negatives. Therefore:

$$\text{Sensitivity} = \frac{\text{number of true positive tests}}{\left(\begin{array}{c}\text{number of true positive tests}\\+\text{number of false negative tests}\end{array}\right)}$$

In the example above, 900 people had true positive tests and 100 had false negative tests. This means that the sensitivity of the exercise test is 900 divided by 900 plus 100, which equals 90%.

Specificity refers to the likelihood of a test being normal (negative) in a population that does NOT have the disease that the test is supposed to detect. For example, if you performed exercise stress tests on 1,000 marathon runners whose coronary arteries were clean as a whistle, you might find that 990 of them have normal test results. However, ten of the tests may be positive (which you know are false positives). In this case, the specificity of exercise stress testing is 99%—the ratio of the true negatives to the sum of the true negatives and the false positives.

$$\text{Specificity} = \frac{\text{number of true negative tests}}{\left(\begin{array}{l}\text{number of true negative tests}\\ +\text{number of false positive tests}\end{array}\right)}$$

Predictive value refers to the likelihood that a positive test indicates the presence of disease. It's defined as the ratio of the true positives to the sum of the true positives and false positives.

$$\begin{array}{l}\text{Predictive value}\\ \text{of a positive test}\end{array} = \frac{\text{number of true positive tests}}{\left(\begin{array}{l}\text{number of true positive tests}\\ +\text{number of false positive tests}\end{array}\right)}$$

No test is 100% sensitive or 100% specific. Every test will have a certain number of false positive or false negative results. Of course, the greater the specificity and sensitivity of a test, the more we can rely on the results.

But another factor comes into play when interpreting diagnostic test results, which is important but often imperfectly understood, even by physicians. This has to do with something called Bayes' Theorem. Bayes was an eighteenth century British clergyman who dabbled in mathematics. To simplify a very complex concept, Bayes' Theorem says that the predictive value of a positive test depends not only on the test's sensitivity and specificity but also on the prevalence of the disease in the population. (**Prevalence** is the number of cases of a disease present in a population at a point in time. **Incidence** is the number of cases of disease occurring over a certain time period, usually a year.) This means that a test is much more apt to give accurate results if it's performed on someone who has a high likelihood of having the disease.

The predictive value of a positive test in a group of people where 50% of them have the disease is very high—90% (assuming the test has a sensitivity and a specificity of 90%). In other words, a positive test in this instance has a lot of predictive value. A person with a positive test is very likely to have the disease. On the other hand, the predictive value of a positive test in a group of people where only 1% has the disease is very low; it falls to 8%. Here's another way to look at it: if a test is performed on someone with very little likelihood of disease, the majority of positive tests will be false positives; in a population with a very high likelihood of disease, the majority of negative tests will be false negatives.

This issue concerning the predictive value of tests comes up time and again with women. Exercise stress tests are sometimes ordered for young premenopausal women who have no risk factors for CAD. The prevalence of disease in this population is so low that the results of exercise stress testing are notoriously misleading. Most positive tests are falsely positive. (The converse holds true for older women, in whom the prevalence of CAD is high. In this group, a negative stress test is likely to be a false negative.) I can't tell you how many young women with no risk factors for CAD have been referred to me over the years for cardiac catheterization because of an "abnormal" stress test. In most cases, I advise the referring physician that a cardiac catheterization isn't necessary. The chances of finding a significant blockage are too remote to justify the small risk of the procedure.

Now that you have some knowledge about the mystifying world of statistics, we can discuss the various diagnostic tests for cardiac disease.

The most commonly ordered test is the electrocardiogram (EKG). In this test, electrodes are placed on the extremities and across the chest to measure the heart's electrical activity from several angles. This information is then displayed graphically on paper over a period of seconds to minutes (FIGURE 8.1).

The heart's electrical impulse normally arises in the sinus node and travels through the atria (the receiving chambers of the heart). This activity generates a deflection on the EKG called the **P wave**. After a short delay, during which the impulse travels through the junction between the atria and the ventricles, the electrical impulse then winds its way through the heart muscle. The deflection caused by the electric current in the ventricles is called the **QRS complex**. The ventricles then recover, or "repolarize," causing the **ST segment** and the T wave of the EKG. Each of these waves, segments, intervals, or deflections provides information about the state of the heart (FIGURE 8.2). Some of the diagnoses that can be made based on an EKG include abnormal heart rhythm,

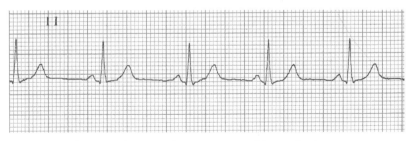

FIGURE 8.1 Electrocardiogram showing a normal heart rhythm.

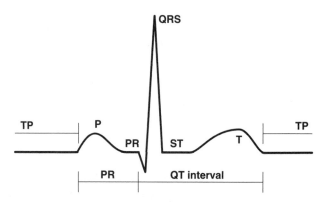

FIGURE 8.2 Diagram of a normal heart rhythm as it appears in an EKG, showing the various components described in the text.

acute or prior heart attack, ischemia, pericarditis, and cardiac enlargement. As discussed earlier, though, no test is 100% sensitive or specific. EKG findings may represent false positives as well as false negatives. In addition, there are some minor differences between the EKGs of men and women. First, women have faster heart rates than men do, and they are more likely to have certain types of tachycardias. Second, the EKG is less sensitive in detecting abnormal thickening of the heart muscle in women than in men.

Perhaps the most likely way an EKG can lead your physician up the garden path is the not infrequent occurrence of errors in performing the test. The electrodes that are attached to the extremities must be put on the proper limb. If any electrodes are switched—for example, if the right and left arm electrodes are accidentally reversed—the EKG will appear to be abnormal. The six chest electrodes also need to be in standard positions. Sometimes large breasts make proper placement of the electrodes difficult. When the chest electrodes aren't placed accurately, the EKG may indicate the presence of a prior heart attack—even in someone who has a completely normal heart. Other causes for misinterpretation include tremors and electrical interference from electronic equipment. Finally, the information derived from the EKG is only as good as the person doing the interpretation. It takes years of training to become skilled in EKG reading, especially in the interpretation of abnormal heart rhythms. The EKG findings must always be correlated with the clinical situation to avoid errors in diagnosis. Falsely labeling someone with cardiac disease may lead to unnecessary, costly, and risky tests as well as a lot of preventable worry and heartache (pun intended).

Stress testing allows your physician to determine how your heart responds when the demands upon it increase. When I was in medical school, we performed a primitive exercise test that involved taking an EKG at rest, having the patient climb up and down a two-step stairway a number of times (depending on his age), then taking another EKG immediately afterwards. This process was called the Master's Test, after the physician who first described its use. A few years later, when I was a cardiology fellow, graded sub-maximal exercise stress testing became common. (It was called sub-maximal because the goal was to have the patient achieve 85% of his or her predicted maximum heart rate.) With this type of test, a person walked on a treadmill or rode a stationary bicycle while hooked up to the EKG machine. In the more common treadmill test, the speed and grade were increased every three minutes until the individual reached a predetermined heart rate that was based on age, or until symptoms occurred. Several EKGs were then performed while the person rested. Physicians looked for characteristic changes in the ST segment. (When the heart is starved for oxygen, the ST segment drops by a millimeter or more from the normal baseline level it occupies when the heart is getting enough oxygen. This finding on the EKG is called ST segment depression.) Unfortunately, there are multiple conditions other than ischemia that can cause ST segment depression, ranging from various drugs to something as simple as hyperventilating. It isn't surprising that the results of exercise stress tests are sometimes misleading. Women have an even higher rate of false positive ST depression than men. We aren't sure why this is so.

Many studies were performed to determine the correlation between exercise stress test results and the findings on coronary angiograms performed in the same patients. It turns out that the more arteries you have blocked, the more sensitive a stress test is. On average, the sensitivity of sub-maximal exercise stress testing is somewhere around 60% to 70%. On the other hand, most studies showed that the specificity of sub-maximal exercise stress testing (the percentage of times the test was negative in individuals who don't have CAD) is about 80% to 90%.

Physicians weren't satisfied with the sensitivity of sub-maximal exercise stress testing and looked for ways to make stress testing more accurate. They also wanted to find a way to stress test the hearts of people who, for whatever reason, couldn't exercise. In response to these challenges, the practice of nuclear stress testing was developed.

In a **nuclear stress test,** you're injected with a radioactive isotope that's distributed to the heart muscle by the coronary arteries. (Radioactive isotopes are chemicals that undergo spontaneous disintegration resulting in the emission of certain types of rays, including x-rays.) After receiving the injection, you're scanned at rest and immediately after exercise by a camera that detects the radiation in the heart. If areas of the heart aren't getting enough blood when you exercise, those areas show up as defects on the scan. Defects that are present both at rest and after exercise usually reflect the presence of scar tissue from a previous heart attack.

The nuclear stress test increased the sensitivity of exercise stress tests to more than 90%. This type of stress test is commonly called a thallium stress test because thallium was one of the earliest isotopes used. Today, thallium's use has been supplanted in many centers by newer isotopes. If you're a woman, your physician may order a Cardiolite nuclear stress test. Cardiolite contains another isotope called technetium, which has higher energy than thallium. Technetium's higher energy decreases the chance of a false positive result, which can result from breast tissue shadowing.

Those who are unable to walk on a treadmill can be offered nuclear stress tests using medications that either dilate blood vessels or increase heart rate and blood pressure. The two most common medications used for this purpose are dipyridamole (Persantine) and dobutamine.

Another, less commonly available form of nuclear test is called a PET scan. Positron emission tomography (PET) is available in some academic centers but not in most hospitals. PET scans can provide information about how metabolically active the heart muscle is. PET scans can help distinguish heart muscle that is injured from heart muscle that is dead. PET scanning can be performed at rest and during exercise to determine in a very accurate fashion whether or not parts of the heart become ischemic with exercise.

When properly carried out, exercise stress testing is very safe. Several years ago, the *Journal of the American Medical Association* reported on 170,000 stress tests. The mortality rate was only 1 in 10,000, which by anyone's standards is a pretty good record. However, care must be taken in performing and interpreting any type of stress test. If you have an unstable pattern of chest pain, uncontrolled congestive heart failure, uncontrolled high blood pressure, or severe narrowing of a heart valve, you shouldn't be subjected to exercise stress testing. Sometimes a myocardial infarction (MI) is caused by a stress test. One study reported that the combined rate of MI and death attributable to exercise stress testing was 1 in 2,500.

Interpreting nuclear scans requires great skill. Artifacts (areas that appear to be abnormal because of factors other than ischemia) can be introduced into the scan by a whole host of factors, most commonly a motion artifact from a patient squirming around while under the camera. The breast can cause shadows on the scan, which causes problems with the interpretation of nuclear stress tests in women, particularly if one of the newer isotopes isn't used. And finally, for any type of stress test, if the target heart rate or other defined endpoint isn't reached, the test is less sensitive.

During the 1990s, another type of exercise test was developed: stress echocardiography. Instead of using a nuclear scan, this test constructs an image of the heart using sound waves. Echocardiography, which is discussed in more detail in the next section, allows physicians to view pictures of the heart beating in real time, without having to open the chest or perform any other invasive procedure. It has truly revolutionized the diagnosis of cardiac disease. By combining exercise with an echocardiogram, we can detect areas of the heart's walls that become sluggish rather than stronger (the normal response of the heart to exercise is to contract more vigorously) with exercise, and thus deduce that the blood supply to that area of the heart is compromised. In people who are unable to exercise, dobutamine can be infused intravenously at increasing doses to stress the heart while echocardiographic images are obtained. This type of test is called a dobutamine stress echo.

My own experience with stress echocardiograms leads me to believe that they are less sensitive than nuclear stress testing in detecting CAD in women. Many women with CAD are overweight, which can interfere with the clarity of the echocardiogram's image. In addition, many women with

CAD are smokers and have chronic lung disease, which also degrades the quality of the image. For these reasons, I usually order a nuclear stress test when I suspect a woman has CAD. If a woman has ST depression on the test but the nuclear scan is normal, then chances are good that she doesn't have significant blockages. However, if a patient has many risk factors and I really think she has CAD, I might decide to recommend a cardiac catheterization, even if the stress test is normal. Over the years I've seen many women who've had several normal stress tests but were found to have significant CAD when they had a heart catheterization.

Given that women develop CAD ten to twenty years later than men do, it isn't surprising that exercise stress testing was thought to be less accurate in women. Remember, the predictive value of a test is lower in a population with a low prevalence of the disease, which is the case for CAD in premenopausal women. So, it's fair to say that stress testing for CAD is less predictive in premenopausal women than it is in men of the same age. However, in older age groups there's no reason to believe that a positive test is less likely to represent a true positive in women than in men.

The echocardiogram is the second most frequently performed cardiac diagnostic test, after the electrocardiogram. Also called a cardiac ultrasound, the echocardiogram is a simple, safe, noninvasive (the body isn't invaded by needles or catheters) test that creates an image of the beating heart using reflected sound waves. The most common is the transthoracic echocardiogram, in which an instrument that produces and measures sound waves is placed in various positions on the chest to generate views of the heart from several angles. Less commonly, your physician will order a **transesophageal echocardiogram** (TEE). In this procedure, you're sedated and you swallow a flexible tube called an endoscope that has the sound transducer located inside it. TEE produces clearer images than a transthoracic echocardiogram because your esophagus (the tube that leads from your mouth to your stomach) butts up against the back of the heart, so there is less distortion and shadowing of the image by chest wall tissue and lung. Obviously, this is a more invasive procedure that involves slight risk from the sedation and the introduction of a foreign object into your body.

Just about any symptom that might be coming from the heart should be investigated with an echocardiogram. People with valvular heart disease should have regular echocardiograms to follow the progression of their disease and aid in the timing of surgery. People with chest pain should have echocardiograms to look for areas of the heart that aren't contracting normally or conditions such as mitral valve prolapse, pericarditis, or the rare cardiac tumor. Patients with hypertension should have echocardiograms to determine if their heart wall is abnormally thick. People with murmurs or suspected congenital heart defects should also have echocardiograms. In short, if your physician sends you to a cardiologist, the chances are good that you will undergo an echocardiogram.

As with any other test, there are pitfalls with echocardiograms. The images may be of poor quality in people with lung disease or obesity. The experience of the technician performing the test and the physician interpreting it plays an important role in how the results are interpreted. Sometimes abnormalities are missed; sometimes minor differences from normal are over-read, generating unnecessary additional testing. For the most part, however, echocardiograms give you and your physician important information about your heart with no risk and little inconvenience.

A Holter monitor is a small, portable device that continuously records an electrocardiogram, usually over a 24-hour period. Your physician will order a Holter monitor if an abnormal heart rhythm (arrhythmia) is suspected or if you faint or complain of frequent palpitations. At times, people have extra beats (premature contractions) without being aware of them. Your physician may also order a Holter monitor based on what appears on your EKG, even if you aren't having symptoms.

It's important that you keep an accurate diary while you are hooked up to the Holter monitor so that any symptoms you have can be correlated with what the EKG looks like at the time. In addition to premature contractions and arrhythmias, a Holter monitor can detect episodes of silent ischemia, instances in which blood supply to the heart muscle is reduced in the absence of symptoms. Of course, there is the chance that your heart may be on its best behavior while the monitor is in place. Just because a Holter monitor is negative (remember, that means it's a positive outcome for you) it doesn't mean that your symptoms aren't coming from the heart. Sometimes several Holter monitors have to be obtained before the diagnosis is clear.

There are also devices called event monitors that you activate only when you're having symptoms, such as palpitations or feelings of dizziness. The EKG signals are then sent over a telephone line to a recording site and transmitted to your physician. Event monitors are most helpful for those people in whom symptoms don't occur on a daily basis. The event monitor is generally kept for a month. In people with infrequent episodes of syncope thought to be due to abnormal heart rhythms, a newer type of event monitor can actually be implanted under the skin. These devices constantly monitor the electrical activity of the heart and record EKGs before, during, and after a fainting spell.

~

Hundreds of thousands of cardiac catheterizations and coronary angiograms are performed in the United States and around the world every year. They remain the "gold standard" for the diagnosis of CAD; they also provide information to surgeons planning valve replacement or repair.

During my early years as a cardiologist, the people who underwent catheterization were admitted to the hospital the night before and kept in the hospital the night of their catheterization. Now, with the advent of managed care and the push to do as much as possible without admitting patients, most cardiac catheterizations are outpatient procedures.

If you're having anginal chest pain despite good medical management and, based on the results of your stress test and knowledge of your risk factors, your doctor feels that you have significant CAD, the chances are that she'll refer you to a cardiologist to have a coronary angiogram. In this procedure, a thin, flexible, hollow tube called a catheter is inserted through an artery (usually the groin artery, the "femoral" artery, but sometimes an arm artery, the "brachial" artery, is used). You're sedated and given a local anesthetic wherever the catheter is to be placed. During the procedure, you lie on a special table in a room equipped with x-ray movie cameras. Your groin or arm is washed off with antiseptic solution to prevent germs from entering the body through the tiny incision made to facilitate the passage of the catheter. Meanwhile, you're hooked up to an EKG that's monitored continuously. The catheter is then connected to a machine that continuously measures your blood pressure. Your blood pressure and your EKG are displayed on a TV screen so that your doctors and nurses can be instantly alerted to any adverse event. Another screen shows the x-ray images of your heart and blood vessels. You may be able to watch this screen, depending on how that particular catheterization laboratory is set up. Throughout the procedure, a device that measures the amount of oxygen in the blood is clipped on your finger. You'll be surrounded by a doctor or two, nurses, and x-ray technicians.

By now you're probably feeling like the star of an epic movie with a cast of thousands. You're feeling no pain from the procedure (or you shouldn't be. If you're feeling pain, something is wrong, and you must let your doctor know right away). After the doctor has manipulated the catheter from the groin up the aorta and into the coronary artery, dye is injected into the artery and x-ray movie pictures of the dye traveling down the artery into the heart muscle are taken. Remember that there are usually two coronary arteries. Each artery has a special catheter that's shaped specifically for it. Each artery must be studied to get a complete picture of the coronary anatomy. Sometimes the dye causes the heart to slow down dramatically, or even stop. This is very anxiety-provoking for your doctor (besides being potentially fatal for you) so all of a sudden your heretofore calm, cool, and collected cath lab team may start screaming "COUGH, COUGH!" at you at the top of their lungs. Obey instantly, and your heart will usually perk right up and start beating at a normal rate. (Coughing helps get the dye out of the heart faster and it's the dye that causes the slowing.)

If your cardiologist is not certain whether plaque buildup in a coronary artery is severe enough to be causing symptoms, she may decide to use a special catheter which can take pictures of the inside of the artery using sound waves. Intravascular ultrasound (IVUS) is a very accurate way to determine the amount of plaque in the arterial wall, and the size of the opening, or lumen, of the artery. Sometimes a plaque that does not appear to be narrowing the artery in the angiogram may, on IVUS, be shown to be causing significant obstruction.

When your doctor is satisfied that enough pictures of the coronary arteries have been taken, he or she may change catheters again and take a picture of the left ventricle as it pumps blood out through the aortic valve into the aorta. This is called a left ventricular angiogram. It usually causes an intense feeling of heat all over the body. In fact, I warn my male patients that they're about to experience what women commonly go through during menopause—a hot flash. (Once when I was a young doctor, an elderly female patient who had just had a left ventricular angiogram exclaimed: "O-o-oh doctor! That made me feel warm in places I haven't felt warm in thirty years!")

After all of the pictures are completed, the catheters are removed and pressure is kept over the artery until there's no bleeding. You then have to lie down for several hours so the newly formed clot that seals the artery isn't dislodged. If all goes well and nothing needs to be corrected immediately you can go home after about six or seven hours.

This is what happens in the course of the usual diagnostic catheterization. Angioplasties are therapeutic procedures utilizing special catheters to open up blocked arteries. They will be discussed in Chapter 10.

When a cardiac catheterization is being performed primarily because of valvular heart disease, your cardiologist also measures pressures in the various chambers of the heart and calculates pressure differences across the valves. She will measure the amount of blood the heart pumps each minute, the cardiac output, and the amount of oxygen in an artery and vein.

A special type of catheterization, called an **electrophysiologic study (EPS)**, is performed for the evaluation of certain abnormal heart rhythms. An EPS study involves putting catheters into the heart and measuring various aspects of its electrical conduction system. At times, abnormal heart rhythms are purposely induced so that medications can be tested for effectiveness. An EPS can be a lengthy procedure, and it's done less commonly than the usual diagnostic catheterization. There are exciting new developments in treatment using catheters to destroy areas of abnormal heart tissue that are causing arrhythmias, but this too will be discussed in Chapter 10.

Computerized tomography (CT) has been used to image the body and diagnose disease since the mid 1970's. This is an x-ray based imaging method in which an x-ray source and detectors rotate around a patient as the patient moves through the scanner. Images are reconstructed from the x-ray data into thin, cross-sectional slices of the body. The impact of CT in clinical medicine has been so profound that its inventors, Sir Godfrey Hounsfield and Allan Cormack, were awarded the 1979 Nobel Prize for Physiology or Medicine. For many years, CT has proven invaluable for diagnosing a variety of diseases related to the blood vessels. These include abnormalities of the aorta such as aneurysms (ballooning) and dissections (tearing of the wall), pulmonary emboli (lung clots), as well as blockages of critical arteries, such as those feeding the brain and kidneys.

Until recently, the relatively small, fast-moving arteries of the heart were beyond the scope of CT imaging. However, substantial technological strides have been made in the past few years and newer generations of CT scanners are now fast enough to freeze the motion of the heart and accurately image the coronary arteries. This type of examination requires the intravenous injection of contrast material, or dye, which is similar to that used in catheter-based angiography and does have a low risk of allergic reaction and kidney damage.

As a novel technique for evaluating the coronary arteries, CT angiography (CTA) is currently receiving a great deal of hype and scrutiny. Studies show that it is a powerful method for non-invasively *excluding* coronary artery disease as a cause of chest pain or positive findings on other studies. If the CT study is normal, then it is highly unlikely that a patient has significant atherosclerotic coronary disease. What is less clear at this point is the accuracy of CTA in grading the severity of any blockages.

CT scanning without the use of dye can also be useful in the evaluation of coronary artery disease. Coronary artery calcium deposits are caused by atherosclerosis. Current CT scanners can quantify the amount of calcium and generate a score that correlates with the overall amount of plaque in a coronary artery but doesn't identify or quantify the degree of coronary narrowing. This technique was established using a largely outmoded type of CT scanner referred to as an Electron beam CT, but has been validated using current scanners.

Another relatively new non-invasive way to obtain information about the heart is called *cardiac MR (CMR)*. The initials MRI stand for magnetic resonance imaging and CMR is a special form of MRI. MRI, like CT, has also had a substantial impact on modern medicine. For their work in the development of MRI, Paul Lauterburg and Peter Mansfield shared the 2003 Nobel Prize for Physiology or Medicine.

MRI has been around as long as angioplasty; both were first performed in humans in 1977. But CMR has only become clinically relevant since about the turn of the millennium. Just as with early CT scans, the use of MRI in detecting heart disease was limited due to the technical challenges of imaging a moving object. However, recent advances in hardware technology and software design have now made it possible to construct highly detailed and accurate pictures of the beating heart.

MRI does not involve any radiation, unlike CTA and cardiac catheterization. Rather, it utilizes strong magnets and radiowaves to detect small, inherent variations in the body's magnetic properties. MRI, like CT, generates thin, cross-sectional images of body structures. The combination of radiofrequency (RF) waves and powerful magnets cause the hydrogen protons in our body's water molecules to vibrate and emit RF energy. MRI scanners detect this emitted energy and convert it into detailed images. (For those who would like a detailed description of how MRI works, a good on-line source of information can be found at *http://www.howstuffworks.com/mri.htm*).

Every disease state is associated with changes in body tissue and because even minor changes in body tissue can affect the rate at which energy is emitted, MRI can detect many diseases at an early stage. In addition to providing a comprehensive, highly accurate evaluation of heart function, CMR also provides information on the extent and severity of heart damage following myocardial infarction. In effect, by delineating the amount of scar in the heart, CMR can tell whether or not surgery or angioplasty will improve heart function after a heart attack. It can very accurately determine the fraction of blood that the heart ejects with each beat (the ejection fraction), and it can detect and characterize masses in the heart, shunt flow across defects, other forms of congenital heart disease, pressure gradients across narrowed valves, and abnormal thickening of the pericardium. Indeed, it is a powerful tool for evaluating a host of cardiac diseases.

Unfortunately, because of the very strong magnets used in MRI, people with metallic implants such as pacemakers, automatic implantable cardiac defribrillators (AICDs) and cochlear implants cannot undergo MR studies.

To improve images, a contrast agent is often used in MRI examinations. The most common is a chemical called gadolinium, which has strong magnetic properties. While most people can tolerate gadolinium-based contrast agents without problem, it is not completely free of adverse reactions. There is a rare disorder called *Nephrogenic Systemic Fibrosis*, (NSF) (also known as nephrogenic fibrosing dermopathy, NFD), which was first described in patients with advanced kidney disease who received gadolinium-based contrast. If a patient is known to have kidney disease, the decision to administer gadolinium must be made judiciously, with careful consideration of the benefits of the MRI study and the severity of the kidney impairment.

Cardiologists would love to have a safe, simple, noninvasive, inexpensive test that would correctly identify every person who has heart disease. Unfortunately, such a test doesn't exist, nor is it likely to in the foreseeable future. So, physicians must make do with the imperfect tests that are available and try to use all of their clinical skills to arrive at the correct diagnosis. Tests must be interpreted in light of everything else your physician knows about you. Putting too much emphasis on one abnormal test result can result in misdiagnosis. I'm reminded of the time my father ran his first half marathon back in the 1970s. He didn't know that distance runners often put Vaseline on pressure points such as the ankles and nipples. By the end of the race his left nipple was abraded to the point that it was bleeding. As he pelted for the finish line, my mother, who was watching, saw the blood and started to scream, "OH MY GOD! THEY SHOT YOUR FATHER!" She was putting too much weight on the finding of blood, and disregarding the fact that he was running at top speed and grinning from ear to ear, findings that would argue against a gunshot wound to the chest.

In summary, there are multiple tests that your cardiologist might order if she suspects that you have cardiac disease. Ideally, she will take a complete history with an emphasis on your symptoms and risk factors and will perform a physical examination of the cardiovascular system. Armed with the knowledge gleaned from this evaluation, your cardiologist may send you back to your primary physician with a clean bill of cardiac health, send you for further testing, or prescribe one or more of the therapies discussed in the next few chapters.

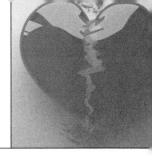

Chapter 9

Medical Therapy for Heart Disease

This chapter introduces you to several types of medications that are used to treat and prevent heart disease. Many of these medicines were discovered or synthesized in the last half of the twentieth century. One exception is digitalis, which is probably the oldest cardiac drug. (For a more extensive look at cardiac medication see my book *Treating and Beating Heart Disease: A Consumer's Guide to Cardiac Medicines*, Jones and Bartlett 2008.)

Digitalis

Digitalis is derived from extracts of the foxglove plant, which was a well-known folk remedy for the "dropsy" in England long before the modern era. This lovely flowering plant carries the Latin name *Digitalis purpurea*, hence the name of the drug. Scientists in our age were able to define the mechanism of action of digitalis and determine why it improves the symptoms of heart failure.

The most commonly prescribed form of digitalis is digoxin (Lanoxin). (Throughout this chapter the generic name for a medicine will be given first, followed by the most common brand name.) Digoxin is used to treat congestive heart failure (CHF) and certain abnormal heart rhythms. It strengthens the contraction of the heart and has important influences on the heart's electrical system. Digitalis was standard first-line therapy for CHF for centuries. It wasn't until the 1990s that a rigorous scientific study was carried out to determine whether digitalis lowered the risk of dying from this condition. In this study, 7,788 people were assigned to receive either digoxin or placebo. No difference in mortality between the treated and placebo groups was found. However, the treated group did require significantly fewer hospitalizations for CHF. When the data were analyzed by gender, it was found that digoxin was less effective in preventing recurrent hospitalizations in women than men. More recently, other studies have seemed to indicate that women treated with digoxin have a higher mortality rate than men. This is probably due to the fact that women are, on average, smaller than men, yet receive the same dose. When the level of digoxin in the blood is kept on the low side, it's likely that women are at no greater risk from this medicine than men.

Digoxin is excreted by the kidneys. Toxic levels of digoxin can build up in people with kidney disease and in the elderly because kidney function declines with age. Because of this potential for build-up, the elderly and people with kidney disease need to take a lower dose of digoxin. When digoxin levels become too high, people feel nauseous and lose their appetite. If you're taking digoxin and develop these side effects, let your physician know immediately. If digitalis levels become too high, there's a significant risk of death.

Diuretics

A diuretic is a medicine that increases the production of urine. Diuretics are used in the treatment of heart failure and high blood pressure. In heart failure, the kidneys retain water and sodium, which eventually leads to swelling or edema. Edema in the lungs causes shortness of breath; edema in the legs causes them to become swollen and uncomfortable. Both can be improved or eliminated by taking diuretics. Furosemide (Lasix) is a commonly prescribed diuretic for CHF.

Many diuretics can cause the body to become depleted of potassium, a blood electrolyte that helps maintain a stable heart rhythm. A commonly prescribed diuretic of this class is hydrochlorothiazide (Esidrix, HydroDIURIL). There are a few diuretics, including spironolactone (Aldactone), eplerenone (Inspra), and triamterene (Dyrenium), which can cause the body to retain potassium. Your physician should check your potassium level periodically if you're taking a diuretic. Abnormally high or abnormally low levels of potassium can be fatal.

If your physician prescribes a diuretic, you may be advised to increase your intake of potassium-rich foods such as oranges and bananas. Alternatively, your physician may prescribe a combination pill that contains a potassium-wasting and a potassium-sparing diuretic. Make sure you discuss these various types of diuretics with your physician so that you're aware of which type you're taking.

ACE Inhibitors

Angiotensin-converting enzyme (ACE) inhibitors are a group of drugs that were developed in the last few decades for the treatment of CHF and high blood pressure. To simplify their very complex mechanism of action, they work by inhibiting an enzyme that's involved in the production of a potent constrictor of blood vessels (hence their name, angiotensin-converting enzyme inhibitor). They also inhibit the breakdown of a blood vessel dilator called bradykinin, allowing the blood vessels to become more relaxed. ACE inhibitors have been proven to decrease the risk of developing kidney disease in diabetics. They can also lessen the burden on the heart in people with leaky heart valves.

Several clinical trials involving many thousands of people have shown that managing CHF with this class of agents prolongs life and decreases the need for hospitalization. Some of the commonly prescribed ACE inhibitors include quinapril (Accupril), enalapril (Vasotec), fosinopril (Monopril), lisinopril (Zestril, Prinivil), capoten (Captopril), benazepril (Lotensin), Moexipril (Univasc), perindopril (Aceon), trandolapril (Mavik), and ramipril (Altace). A dry cough is the most frequent side effect of ACE inhibitors. Women are two to three times more likely to develop cough than men. Less commonly, an allergic reaction characterized by swelling of the mouth, lips, tongue, and larynx can occur. This swelling can be fatal. Rarely, the white blood cell count can fall to abnormal levels in patients taking ACE inhibitors. This is more likely to happen in people with kidney disease. People with kidney disease are also more likely to experience some worsening of their kidney function tests and abnormal elevations of blood potassium levels. At times, blood pressure can drop to dangerously low levels when using ACE inhibitors, so be sure to tell your physician if you feel dizzy or faint while taking this type of medicine. Pregnant women should never take ACE inhibitors because they can cause injury and even death to the fetus.

Angiotensin Receptor Blockers (ARBs)

ARBs are medicines which block the action of Angiotensin II, a chemical made in the kidney which causes the smooth muscle in arteries to constrict, thereby raising blood pressure. They are used in the treatment of high blood pressure and congestive heart failure. They are also used to delay the progression of kidney disease in diabetics. They are less likely than ACE inhibitors to cause a cough or allergy but may cause high blood levels of potassium, worsening kidney failure and, harm or death to a fetus. They include candesartan (Atacand), eprosartan (Teveten), irbesartan (Avapro), losartan (Cozaar), olmesartan (Benicar), telmisartan (Micardis), and valsartan (Diovan).

Beta-Blockers

When I was an intern, beta-blockers were a new class of medicine that had just won approval from the Food and Drug Administration (FDA). Beta-blockers block the action of the sympathetic nervous system, which activates the "fight or flight" response. They lower pulse rate whether a person is at rest or exercising and they lower blood pressure.

We used to believe that beta-blockers were dangerous in people with CHF, but now we have evidence that treatment with beta-blockers actually improves cardiac function and prolongs life in people with CHF. They are also useful in treating certain abnormal heart rhythms and have been shown to lower the likelihood of sudden cardiac death. Beta-blockers are standard therapy in people with coronary artery disease (CAD), in whom they cause a marked reduction in the frequency of angina. Some of the commonly prescribed beta-blockers are metoprolol (Lopressor and Toprol), propranolol (Inderal), atenolol (Tenormin), nadolol (Corgard), carvedilol (Coreg), labetolol (Normodyne, Trandate), and bisoprolol (Zebeta). In late 2007, the FDA approved nebivolol (Bystolic) for the treatment of high blood pressure.

Fatigue is the most common side effect of beta-blockers, but it occurs in less than 10% of patients. People with asthma may develop increased wheezing with beta-blockers, so their use is generally avoided in asthmatics. Depression and dizziness may occur. Beta-blockers can also mask the symptoms of low blood glucose. They may cause elevated triglyceride levels and may exacerbate pain in the legs in patients with blockages in the arteries supplying the lower extremities. Despite these potential side effects, most people have no problem taking beta-blockers and they save lives.

People with CAD shouldn't stop taking beta-blockers abruptly. Doing so can cause worsening angina and heart attacks. Propranolol, the first beta-blocker approved by the FDA, has been reported to cause erectile dysfunction in rare instances. In general however, beta-blockers are safe and well tolerated. Unless there are strong reasons not to be, everyone who has heart failure or CAD should be treated with a beta-blocker.

Nitrates

Angina pectoris is usually the first symptom that women experience when they develop CAD. However, unlike the classic mid-chest pressure that men typically complain of, women are apt to experience angina pectoris in other locations, such as the jaw, back, neck, and shoulders. The first medicine that was shown to be of benefit in relieving angina pectoris was nitroglycerin. It was first synthesized in 1846. By 1879 the British physician William Murrell established that taking nitroglycerin under the tongue (what doctors call sublingual nitroglycerin) could relieve angina pectoris and could prevent attacks when taken prophylactically.

Nitroglycerin belongs to a class of drugs called organic nitrates, several of which are used to treat angina pectoris. They work by dilating blood vessels and decreasing the work of the heart. When I prescribe nitroglycerin, I always tell my patients that they may get a headache. This is a good sign because it indicates that the medicine is working (dilation of the vessels in the brain can cause a headache). I also tell my patients to take the first dose sitting down because nitroglycerin can cause a sudden drop in blood pressure, which, if severe enough, can cause dizziness and even fainting. Sitting makes this less likely, and if you get dizzy while you're sitting, you're less likely to fall.

The effect of nitroglycerin taken under the tongue is short, varying from about 10 to 30 minutes. When nitroglycerin is taken through the skin, in the form of a patch or paste, the duration of action can be several hours. Some longer acting nitrates used in the treatment of angina include isosorbide (Isordil), a pill taken orally, nitroglycerin patches, and nitroglycerin paste.

Ranolazine

In January 2006, the FDA approved a new medicine for the treatment of angina.

Ranolazine (trade name Ranexa) does not work by relaxing blood vessels or decreasing pulse or blood pressure. In fact, researchers are not sure why it is effective in lowering the frequency of anginal attacks, but it appears to work at the level of the cardiac muscle cell to improve the efficiency of oxygen utilization. It should be used in people who are already receiving nitrates, beta-blockers, and calcium channel blockers (CCBs) but are still significantly limited by angina. Although effective in women, ranolazine seems to have less of an effect on angina frequency and exercise tolerance in women compared to men. In addition, there is no evidence that treatment with ranolazine decreases the risk of heart attack or death in men or women. Ranolazine can prolong something called the QT interval, a finding on the EKG. Prolongation of the QT interval can increase the risk of abnormal heart rhythms so people with this finding should not take ranolazine. The blood levels of certain medicines, including simvastatin and digoxin, may increase when ranolazine is taken, so their dosages should be reduced.

Calcium Channel Blockers

The **calcium channel blockers** came into common use in the 1980s in the United States. Before then, this group of medications had been in use in Europe for many years. Calcium channel blockers work by dilating blood vessels and lowering blood pressure. In fact, they are commonly prescribed to treat hypertension in addition to angina. Some of the calcium channel blockers also slow the heart rate, and are useful in people who can't tolerate beta-blockers, such as those with asthma. The short-acting forms of certain calcium channel blockers were associated with increased mortality when they were given to patients with unstable angina. Nowadays, most people who take these medicines take a long-acting preparation. Diltiazem (Cardizem, **Dilacor, Tiazac**), verapamil (**Calan, Covera, Isoptin**), amlodipine (Norvasc), nifedipine (**Procardia,** Adalat), and felodipine (Plendil) are names of some of the commonly prescribed calcium channel blockers. Constipation can be a side effect, particularly of verapamil. Sometimes swelling of the ankles occurs with the certain calcium channel blockers, including amlodipine, nifedipine, and felodipine; this side effect is more likely to occur in women. If verapamil or diltiazem are used together with beta-blockers, the pulse can become dangerously slow. This is more likely to occur in the elderly.

Other High Blood Pressure Medicines

Alpha-blockers are a class of medicines that relax blood vessels, leading to a lowering of the blood pressure. Examples of alpha-blockers include terazosin (Hytrin), prazosin (Minipress), and doxazosin (Cardura). The most common side effect of alpha-blockers is dizziness, which can be severe enough to causing fainting. Other common side effects include headache and palpitations.

There is another class of older high blood pressure medicines called "centrally acting drugs" because they are thought to affect the central nervous system. The only one of this class of medicine that is used commonly today is clonidine (Catapres). It can cause drowsiness, dry mouth, and erectile dysfunction. Clonidine should not be stopped abruptly because doing so can cause a dangerous increase in blood pressure.

There are also drugs which are considered direct "vasodilators." These include hydralazine (Apresoline) and minoxidil (Loniten). They can cause flushing, headache, fluid retention, and in the case of minoxidil excess hair growth (hence its use applied to the head as a salve called Rogaine in balding). Hydralazine has a rare but potentially serious side effect in that it has been implicated in the development of a disease called *lupus erythematosis*, a disorder in which the body attacks its own tissue. Minoxidil can cause severe drops in blood pressure so it is not used except in rare instances when blood pressure cannot be controlled by other means.

In 2007, the FDA approved a new medicine to treat high blood pressure. Called aliskiren (Tekturna), it works by blocking the action of a naturally occurring hormone produced by the kidneys called renin, which causes arteries to constrict, thereby leading to high blood pressure. Aliskiren appears to be less effective in lowering blood pressure in blacks than whites but has few side effects, the most frequent being diarrhea.

Your physician may need to prescribe multiple medications to bring your pressure down to a healthy range, particularly if you're older or if your blood pressure is severely elevated. With so many medications available, your physician should be able to find a combination that's effective and well tolerated.

Medicines for Primary Pulmonary Hypertension (PPH)

People with this condition are usually treated with the blood thinner warfarin (Coumadin) and a calcium channel blocker like amlodipine (Norvasc) or nifedipine (Procardia). However there are newer, more effective medicines for this condition, including intravenous medicines, a medicine taken as a nasal spray, and some oral medicines. The intravenous medicine is called epoprostenol (Flolan). The nasal spray is iloprost (Ventavis). The oral medications include bosentan (Tracleer), ambrisentan (Letairis), and sildenafil (Revatio). The last is perhaps better known as Viagra, a medicine used to treat erectile dysfunction which was serendipitously found to improve PPH. With the exception of sildenafil, the use of these oral medicines is strictly controlled because of the risk of serious side effects, mainly liver damage and the risk of fetal harm in pregnant women. They are available only through a restricted distribution program in centers specializing in the treatment of PPH.

Aspirin and Similar Medicines

In Europe, extracts of willow bark were used to treat fever for centuries. The Latin name for the white willow is Salix alba vulgaris. The class of compounds derived from willow was named salicylates. The active ingredient of willow bark was first isolated in 1827 and was named salicin. Aspirin, whose chemical name is acetylsalicylic acid, was introduced in 1899.

Platelets are small elements in the blood that are important in the formation of clots. Aspirin interferes with the ability of platelets to aggregate or clump, which they must do if a clot is to form. Aspirin, therefore, lowers the risk of a clot forming when a plaque ruptures. As little as 81 mg of aspirin, the dose in a baby aspirin, inhibits platelets from clumping for 72 hours. At higher doses, aspirin can also dilate blood vessels and combat inflammation. All of these favorable effects explain the usefulness of aspirin in the treatment of atherosclerosis.

There are other platelet inhibitors that have been studied for their effect on heart attacks, strokes, and cardiovascular death. Many studies involving thousands of people have demonstrated that aspirin and the other antiplatelet medications lower the risk of cardiovascular events in people who have atherosclerosis. This benefit extends to women as well as men. When the data from many antiplatelet trials were pooled in 1988, investigators found a 32% reduction in nonfatal heart attacks, a 27% reduction in stroke, and a 15% reduction in mortality in 29,000 patients with a documented history of cardiovascular disease. In 1994, another review confirmed similar findings in more than 40,000 patients. Unfortunately, women are still less likely than men to be treated with aspirin after a heart attack.

Other studies involving mainly men proved that low dose aspirin is effective in lowering men's risk of heart attack even when given to healthy men who had no apparent atherosclerosis. Whether aspirin could lower the risk of heart attack or stroke in women without atherosclerosis was not known until the results of the Women's Health Study of aspirin were published in 2005. This study enrolled more than 27,000 healthy women age 45 or older who were treated with either 100 mg of aspirin every other day or placebo. In women who took aspirin there was no decrease in their risk of heart attack but the risk of stroke was reduced by 17%. When the results for women who were 65 or older at entry into the study were analyzed, these older women reduced their risk of heart attack by 34% and stroke by 30%. However, even this low dose increased the risk of serious bleeding, in women on aspirin compared to women on placebo. There was no difference in the death rate between women on aspirin or placebo. The bottom line is that unless there is a very strong reason not to take aspirin, all women with diagnosed cardiovascular disease, and healthy women who are 65 years of age or older should take low dose aspirin. For women between the ages of 45 and 64, the risk of bleeding must be weighed against the 17% reduction in the risk of stroke.

Some of the other antiplatelet medications are ticlopidine (Ticlid), dipyridamole (Persantine), and clopidogrel (Plavix). All can be used in combination with aspirin. All, like aspirin, are associated with an increased risk of hemorrhage.

Anticoagulants

If you have an artificial heart valve or have a common abnormal heart rhythm called atrial fibrillation, chances are you're taking the medication warfarin (Coumadin). You probably didn't know that you were taking rat poison! Warfarin makes it harder for blood to clot by inhibiting the body's ability to manufacture certain clotting factors that depend on the action of Vitamin K. It takes a few days, sometimes three or four, for the full anti-clotting effect of warfarin to occur. When you're taking this medicine, your physician will order blood tests on a regular basis to be sure your blood is neither too thick nor too thin. Sometimes people on warfarin are told to avoid foods rich in Vitamin K such as green leafy vegetables, but I believe this is wrong! Eating many different kinds of vegetables has benefits that far outweigh the effect of Vitamin K on clotting factors. I tell my patients to eat a healthy diet and that I will adjust their dose as needed.

It helps to avoid radical changes in diet while taking warfarin. Any illness associated with vomiting or diarrhea should be reported to your physician so your blood tests can be monitored more closely and your dose can be adjusted, if necessary. Many other medications can interfere with or strengthen the effect of warfarin, so be sure any health care provider you see knows every medicine you're currently taking before he or she prescribes a new one. Women who are pregnant shouldn't take warfarin except for very limited indications because it has been reported to cause fatal hemorrhage and is associated with congenital malformations. Finally, switching from the brand Coumadin to a generic preparation of warfarin may throw your blood work off. Be sure your pharmacist always fills your prescription with the same brand.

Thrombolytics: The "Clot Busters"

You've read several times that most heart attacks are caused when plaque in a coronary artery ruptures and a clot forms in the area of rupture. If the clot totally obstructs the artery, the heart muscle beyond that point will usually die from lack of oxygen.

During the 1980s, thousands of people in the throes of a heart attack were treated with a new class of agents called thrombolytics (also called "clot busters"). These drugs work by dissolving clots, thereby restoring blood flow. Women made up 20% to 27% of the participants in these clinical trials. Some of the data obtained from these trials showed that the mortality benefit was less for women than men. Other studies showed no significant difference in mortality rates between men and women. However, just about all of these studies showed that women—particularly elderly women—were more likely to suffer the most dreaded complication of thrombolytics: bleeding into the brain. Women are two to three times more likely than men to have a brain hemorrhage after receiving a clot buster. Bleeding elsewhere in the body is also more common in women. For this reason I feel strongly that other methods for restoring blood flow (for example angioplasty, which is discussed in detail in the next chapter) should be the first choice to treat heart attacks in older women. In fact, I have asked every cardiologist I know at one time or another whether he or she would prefer to be treated with thrombolytics or angioplasty if they were having a heart attack. I have yet to hear a cardiologist choose the clot buster over angioplasty.

Unfortunately, many people don't live near a hospital that has a cardiac catheterization laboratory, whereas any hospital can provide thrombolytics. So, if there are no reasons that would make thrombolytics too risky (what physicians call a *contraindication*), and an angioplasty isn't in the offing, people in the throes of a heart attack should receive a clot buster. Situations in which the use of a clot buster is too risky include uncontrolled high blood pressure, a history of stroke, recent surgery, and active bleeding (except for menstrual bleeding). Although only small numbers of menstruating women have received these drugs, they appear to be safe in this situation.

Heparin

Heparin is a drug that inhibits blood clotting by a different mechanism than aspirin. It's standard therapy for heart attacks and unstable angina. It can be given directly into a vein. Alternatively, another form of heparin, called enoxaparin (Lovenox), can be injected into the skin.

IIb/IIIa Inhibitors

Another class of antiplatelet drugs is called IIb/IIIa inhibitors. They are commonly given to patients who are having an angioplasty. They are also given to certain high-risk patients with unstable angina. Some examples of this class of medicine are abciximab (ReoPro) and eptifibatide (Integrilin).

Statins and Other Medicines for High Blood Fats

Statins are a class of medicines that have proven to be life saving for people with atherosclerosis. Thousands of people have participated in secondary prevention trials to determine if treatment with statins lowers the death rate, and the rate of heart attack or other vascular events, in people with coronary artery disease. There have also been three primary prevention trials that studied the effect of statins on cardiovascular events in people without diagnosed coronary artery disease but only two of these included women.

One of the largest secondary prevention trials was the Heart Protection Study, which involved more than 20,000 people who had either diagnosed vascular disease or diabetes. The results of this trial were published in the British medical journal, *The Lancet*, in July, 2002. The study participants were randomly assigned to either placebo or simvastatin (Zocor). The primary outcomes were death from any cause and fatal and non-fatal vascular events. 25% of the participants were women. The Heart Protection Study found that treatment with simvastatin significantly reduced deaths from all causes, deaths due to coronary disease, fatal and nonfatal strokes, and nonfatal heart attacks. The treated group also had a much lower likelihood of needing a revascularization procedure like angioplasty or bypass surgery. These beneficial results were seen in both women and men and across the age range of the participants—40 to 80 years.

An interesting feature of the Heart Protection Study is that antioxidants were also studied in a randomized, double-blind fashion. In addition to either simvastatin or placebo, all of the participants in this trial received an indistinguishable placebo or a pill containing 600 mg of Vitamin E, 250 mg of Vitamin C, and 20 mg of beta-carotene a day. When the results were analyzed, there was no difference in the antioxidant treated versus placebo treated participants in deaths from any cause, or deaths due to vascular disease. Nor was there a difference in the numbers of people who had heart attacks, fatal or nonfatal strokes, or revascularization. There was also no significant difference in the incidence of cancers between the two groups.

Other secondary prevention trials demonstrated similar results. The Cholesterol and Recurrent Events (CARE) trial involved more than 4,000 people (3,583 men and 576 women) who had suffered a heart attack within 3 to 20 months before being enrolled in the study. Half were treated with pravastatin (Pravachol) and half were given a placebo. The study found an overall reduction of 24% in the risk of nonfatal heart attack and coronary heart disease death. There was also a significant reduction in the need for bypass surgery or angioplasty in the people treated with pravastatin. The beneficial results in this study applied to women as well as men. In fact women had a greater reduction in risk than men in this trial. Women had a 43% reduction in the risk of death from CHD or nonfatal heart attack compared to a 21% reduction for men. Strokes were reduced by 56% in women treated with pravastatin and were reduced by 25% in men, compared to women and men given the placebo. The subjects in this study did not have strikingly elevated cholesterol levels; the improvement in cholesterol levels was similar in men and women.

Two other secondary prevention trials with statins deserve to be mentioned. Both of these studies compared intensive statin treatment with less intensive statin treatment. The first to be reported, in 2004, was called the PROVE-IT TIMI 22 study. It compared outcomes in over 4,000 people (22% were women) who were having unstable coronary symptoms, what doctors call an "acute coronary syndrome" or ACS. Half received 80 mg/day of atorvastatin and half received 40 mg/day of pravastatin. The people in the former group achieved an average LDL cholesterol of 65 mg/dl; the people in the latter group achieved an average LDL cholesterol of 92 mg/dl. After a mean follow-up period of 24 months, those treated more intensively had a relative risk reduction for major cardiovascular events of 16% compared to those treated less intensively, and this benefit was statistically significant in both men and women. (When a result is said to be "statistically significant" it means that the results are very likely due to the treatment and very unlikely due to chance.)

The second study was called the Treatment to New Targets trial, and it involved just over 10,000 people with stable CAD of whom 19% were women. The results of this study were first reported in 2005. Half of the people in this trial were treated with 80 mg a day of atorvastatin and half were treated with 10 mg a day of the same drug. The former group achieved an average LDL cholesterol of 77 mg/dl and the latter achieved an average cholesterol of 101 mg/dl. There was a 22% relative risk reduction for major cardiovascular events in the intensively treated group. In this trial also, the benefit was statistically significant in women as well as men.

When it comes to primary prevention trials the data for women are not so clear. The first primary prevention study which included women was the Air Force/Texas Coronary Atherosclerosis Prevention Study (AFCAPS/TexCAPS). 5,608 men and 997 women with average levels of total and LDL cholesterol, below average levels of HDL cholesterol, and no evidence of atherosclerosis were treated with lovastatin (Mevacor) or placebo. The primary endpoints were fatal or nonfatal heart attack, unstable angina, or sudden cardiac death. Among men there were 109 primary events in the lovastatin group and 170 primary events in the placebo group. This was a statistically significant reduction. Among women there were 7 primary events in the lovastatin group and 13 primary events in the placebo group. Because there were so few events in women, this difference was not statistically significant.

The other primary prevention trial that enrolled women was the Anglo-Scandinavian Cardiac Outcomes Trial-Lipid Lowering Arm (ASCOT-LLA). Men and women between the ages of 40 and 79 who had high blood pressure and at least three other cardiac risk factors were randomized to receive either atorvastatin (Lipitor) or placebo in addition to medicine to lower blood pressure. Out of 10,305 people enrolled in the cholesterol lowering part of this trial, 1,942 (19%) were women. The primary endpoints were nonfatal heart attack and death due to coronary heart disease. The trial was stopped prematurely because 100 primary events had occurred in the atorvastatin group compared to 154 events in the placebo group after a little over three years. There was also a significant reduction in the number of strokes in the people treated with atorvastatin. When the study results were analyzed only for the women there was no statistically significant benefit of statin treatment in women. In fact there were 19 primary endpoint events in women treated with atorvastatin and 17 events in the women on placebo.

In men, the event rate in these two primary prevention trials was lowered from 4.4% to 2.7%, a difference that was significant. In women the event rate was lowered from 2.1% to 1.8%, which was not significant. In the first five large secondary prevention trials mentioned above, which enrolled over 43,000 people with established vascular disease, the event rate for men was lowered from 25.5% to 19.5%. In women in these five studies the event rate was decreased from 17% to 13.9%. Both men and women with cardiovascular disease had significant benefit from statins in these studies. The bottom line is that we know that statin medications are effective in the primary prevention of atherosclerotic cardiovascular disease in men. It is possible that statin therapy is effective for primary prevention of atherosclerotic cardiovascular disease in women but we cannot be certain of this. What we can say is that in women with established cardiovascular disease, there is no doubt that statins lower the risk of coronary and other vascular events. They just don't work as well in women as they do in men.

The statins work by inhibiting an enzyme involved in the manufacture of cholesterol by the body. Statins also appear to have an anti-inflammatory effect. They lower the other major blood fat, triglycerides, by a modest amount. Lovastatin (Mevacor), atorvastatin (Lipitor), fluvastatin (Lescol), pravastatin (Pravachol), and simvastatin (Zocor) are the commonly prescribed statins in the United States. In 2003 a new statin, rosuvastatin (Crestor) was approved by the Food and Drug Administration. On average, you can expect that taking one of these medicines will cause a 25% to 60% reduction in your LDL cholesterol, a 5% to 14% increase in your HDL cholesterol, and a 10% to 25% drop in your triglycerides.

Although these drugs have an excellent safety record, there are two possible side effects that your doctor should discuss with you before starting a statin. In about 1% of people treated with statins, abnormalities of liver function tests occur. For this reason you should have a liver function blood test before starting therapy, 12 weeks after starting therapy, whenever the dose is increased and about every 6 months thereafter. If the test is more than 3 times the upper limit of normal, your dose will be decreased or the medication will be stopped. Patients with active liver disease should not be treated with statins, and they should be used with caution in patients who consume substantial quantities of alcohol.

A more serious potential side effect is myopathy or myositis, which is defined as muscle aches or weakness in conjunction with elevations in an enzyme called creatine phosphokinase (CPK). CPK is found in both cardiac and skeletal muscle and is released into the blood stream when there is muscle damage. You need to notify your physician if you develop muscle pain or weakness while taking a statin, especially if the muscle pain is diffuse, or associated with fever or dark urine. The latter occurs when large amounts of muscle breakdown products are presented to the kidneys and this abrupt load on the kidneys can cause them to fail. The risk of this complication is increased if you take certain other medicines while you are on a statin, so be sure to give every physician you see a list of any medicine you are taking. The medicines that have been implicated in statin induced muscle damage include cyclosporine (a drug used in patients who have had organ transplants), certain antifungal antibiotics like Sporanox, erythromycin, niacin, and another class of lipid lowering medicine called fibric acid derivatives. Impaired kidney function also increases the risk of this complication. Remember that not every ache or pain you feel if you are taking a statin will be caused by the medicine. Muscle damage is a very rare complication of statins. When in doubt, call your doctor and let her examine you and get blood tests to see if your symptoms are due to the medicine or have some other cause. Statins can be life saving and should not be stopped without good cause. I also tell my patients that they may feel flu-like symptoms for the first several days after starting a statin. Again, this is nothing to be alarmed about and not a reason to stop the medication. The feeling almost always subsides in a few days.

Women of childbearing age should be cautioned that statins may cause harm to the fetus if they become pregnant. They should be used only when a woman does not plan on becoming pregnant, and if pregnancy occurs, the statin should be discontinued.

Fibric Acid Derivatives

The first line of therapy for people with a high triglyceride level (which is usually associated with low HDL cholesterol) is weight loss. Because smoking raises triglycerides and lowers HDL, it goes without saying that smokers must quit. Reducing alcohol intake is also important because alcohol can cause marked elevations in triglycerides. Your physician should do blood tests to be certain that you don't have diabetes or an underactive thyroid, two conditions that can elevate triglycerides. Certain drugs, including beta-blockers and thiazide diuretics, can cause significant increases in triglyceride levels in patients with familial diseases that raise triglycerides. And finally, some women with these familial disorders develop very high levels when given estrogen, either in the form of oral contraceptives or as hormone replacement therapy after menopause. Before prescribing medicines your physician should be certain that you aren't taking medications or have a disease that might be causing the increase in your blood fats.

If after the above measures are taken your triglycerides remain elevated, your physician may prescribe one of the fibric acid derivatives. These include clofibrate (Atromid), gemfibrozil (Lopid), and fenofibrate (Tricor). Clofibrate and gemfibrozil have little effect on LDL levels but increase HDL cholesterol by 5% to 15% and lower triglycerides by 25% to 40%. Fenofibrate, the most recent fibric acid derivative to be approved by the FDA, lowers total and LDL cholesterol levels in addition to lowering triglycerides and raising HDL cholesterol.

The fibric acid derivatives cause an increased incidence of gallstones and have also been shown to cause elevations in liver enzymes and, rarely, muscle damage. Clofibrate (Atromid) was the first of these drugs to be approved by the FDA. Two large-scale studies of clofibrate didn't show a convincing reduction in the incidence of fatal heart attacks in the treated group, and in one study the treated group had a significantly higher mortality due to non-cardiac causes. One of the studies found that there was a higher rate of abnormal heart rhythms in the group given clofibrate. Because of these safety concerns, there is only one indication for using clofibrate and that is for a rare disease called Type III hyperlipidemia.

The second fibric acid derivative to be approved by the FDA was gemfibrozil (Lopid). It is indicated to treat patients with very high (above 500 mg/dl) triglycerides who don't respond to dietary treatment or to treat patients who have elevated LDL and triglycerides combined with low HDL. Gemfibrozil was shown to reduce heart attacks and coronary death in men with a history of coronary disease but this study was done in Veteran's Administration hospitals and it didn't include women. Whether women would also benefit from gemfibrozil therapy isn't known, but because a low HDL level is the lipid abnormality that most strongly predicts cardiac events in women older than age 65, such a study would be very useful.

Fenofibrate (Tricor), the latest fibric acid derivative to be approved, is used to treat people with elevations in triglycerides levels. Fenofibrate has also been approved to treat elevations in LDL cholesterol and low levels of HDL cholesterol. In a large study of almost 10,000 people with adult-onset diabetes there was an 11% reduction in the risk of total cardiovascular disease events in those treated with fenofibrate compared to placebo. The diabetic patients treated with fenofibrate in this study (called the FIELD trial) also had lower rates of amputations and laser treatment for diabetic eye disease.

Fibric acid derivatives should not be taken by pregnant or nursing women. All three of the medicines described above can cause bleeding complications in people taking warfarin (Coumadin). Once again, I want to emphasize that every physician who prescribes a medicine for you must be informed of every other drug you're taking.

Bile Acid Sequestrants

The first medicines used to treat elevations in cholesterol were the bile acid sequestrants. Bile acids form from cholesterol. They help in the digestion and absorption of fats. By binding to bile acids, the sequestrants increase the excretion of bile acids and cause serum cholesterol and LDL cholesterol levels to decrease. Cholestyramine (Questran), colestipol (Colestid), and colesevelam (Welchol) are examples of this type of medication. Constipation and increased flatulence (the fancy medical term for the common fart) are the major side effects of these medicines. They need to be taken two to three times per day. The early preparations were powders that had a gritty consistency and had to be mixed with liquid. Today, Colestid and Welchol come in tablet form and are easier to take. These medicines are considered very safe because they aren't absorbed into the body. They can be taken in conjunction with statins without increasing the risk of liver or muscle damage. Some patients treated with bile acid sequestrants will develop elevated triglyceride levels.

Zetia

The newest medicine to treat high cholesterol is ezetimibe (Zetia). This is the first truly new class of anti-cholesterol medicine to come along in decades. Ezetimibe blocks the absorption of cholesterol from the bowel and has few side effects, the most common being fatigue and diarrhea in about 2 to 4 percent of those who take it. Allergic reactions in the form of a rash have also been reported. It can be used alone or in combination with a statin. When taken alone, it lowers total cholesterol by about 15% and LDL cholesterol by about 20%. Studies are underway to determine if adding ezetimibe to a statin lowers the risk of cardiac events when used with a statin, compared to statin therapy alone. These studies are expected to be completed in 2010.

Niacin

Niacin is one of the B vitamins (B_3). It does everything you'd want a lipid-lowering agent to do. It lowers triglycerides by 25% to 35%, lowers LDL cholesterol by 15% to 25%, and raises HDL cholesterol by 15% to 30%. No other agent has such a potent effect on HDL cholesterol levels. Unfortunately, it has several side effects that limit its use. It must be given in doses of 1 to 2 grams per day, which is many times higher than the minimum daily adult requirement. When taken in such high doses, niacin usually causes intense flushing and itching. This can sometimes be avoided by starting with a low dose and increasing it gradually or by pretreatment with aspirin. A timed release form of niacin, called Niaspan, has a much lower likelihood of causing flushing.

Niacin can also cause liver damage and can cause acute attacks of gout by raising the level of uric acid in the blood. In addition, it can elevate blood glucose levels in diabetics or in those prone to diabetes.

Treatment with niacin in men with CAD has been shown to lower the incidence of nonfatal heart attacks. It has also been shown to decrease the rate of progression of plaque in coronary arteries, and lessen the amount of plaque in treated people. Unfortunately, there weren't enough women included in these studies to be certain that the beneficial results extend to women. However, a study currently underway called the AIM-HIGH trial is comparing simvastatin plus niacin to simvastatin plus placebo in more than 3,000 men and women with vascular disease, high triglycerides, and low HDL cholesterol. This study will determine if adding niacin to statin can further reduce risk in people with vascular disease. Results are expected in 2011.

At any given dose, niacin appears to have a greater effect on lipids in women than men. It can be combined safely with fibric acid derivatives and bile acid sequestrants. It can be taken in conjunction with statins as long as there is careful monitoring for side effects. Patients on niacin should have their liver function tests monitored at the same frequency as those taking statins.

Fish Oils

Fish oils, which contain large amounts of omega-3 fatty acids, lower triglyceride levels. The therapeutic dose is 2 to 4 grams a day, which requires the ingestion of several capsules per day, depending on the number of grams in each capsule. There is an FDA approved prescription omega-3 fatty acid medicine called Lovaza, which is a highly purified preparation of fish oils. It comes in 1,000 mg capsules and the usual dose is three to four a day. It is indicated in people who have triglyceride levels of more than 500 mg/dl.

If you're taking fish oils, be prepared to smell like a tuna fish sandwich. An alternative is to eat fish at least twice a week. The fish that provide the greatest amount of omega-3 fatty acids include salmon, herring, mackerel, and trout. Walnuts are another good source, but they have more calories per unit of weight than fish do. As we noted earlier, the American Heart Association recommends that people with diagnosed cardiovascular disease take fish oil supplements in a dose of 3 grams per day.

Treatment of Abnormal Heart Rhythms

If you have an abnormally fast heart rate (called tachycardia), your physician will obtain blood tests to rule out an overactive thyroid. The medications available to treat tachycardias are divided into four classes. Two of these have already been discussed, beta-blockers (Class II) and the calcium channel blockers verapamil and diltiazem (Class IV). In addition, digitalis has long been used to slow the heart rate in people with atrial fibrillation. In atrial fibrillation, the atria (the upper chambers of the heart) beat rapidly and irregularly. The ventricles beat at a slower rate than the atria, but usually at a rate that's uncomfortably fast for the person experiencing this arrhythmia. Blood tends to stagnate in the fibrillating atria, and they lose the ability to contract normally. This predisposes to the formation of clots, which can break off and travel to the brain and cause a stroke. For this reason, most people with atrial fibrillation are treated with the blood thinner warfarin (Coumadin). Blood thinners, or **anticoagulants**, are also given to people who have artificial heart valves and to some patients after a stroke or heart attack.

Class I drugs decrease the excitability of the heart. They include lidocaine, procainamide (Pronestyl), quinidine (Quinidex), disopyramide (Norpace), and flecainide (Tambocor). In addition to stopping tachycardias, these medications sometimes actually cause a tachycardia called "torsade de pointes" (as can Class III drugs). This complication occurs more commonly in women than men. It can lead to cardiac arrest. When it occurs the drug that is thought to be responsible is stopped.

Class III drugs include amiodarone (Cordarone) and dofetilide (Tikosyn). Sotalol (Betapace) is a drug that has beta-blocking and Class III properties. Amiodarone, dofetilide, and sotalol are useful for preventing atrial fibrillation.

Because of the incidence of serious side effects with all of these medicines and the lack of good evidence of a beneficial effect on mortality (except for beta-blockers and amiodarone), the treatment of tachycardias has undergone a revolution. Catheter-based therapies and devices called **automatic implantable cardiac defibrillators (AICDs)** are now being used more and more often to treat arrhythmias. These devices are discussed in the next chapter.

There are dozens of medications that your physician can prescribe to prevent heart disease or to alleviate symptoms and prolong life if you have heart disease. Many have been introduced in the last few decades, and newer drugs are coming on the market all the time. It's vital that you take such medicines as prescribed. You also need to inform every doctor or nurse practitioner you see of every medicine you're taking, even if it's an over-the-counter preparation. Many medicines interact with each other and can increase the likelihood of side effects when taken together. Don't stop taking a medicine without informing your physician. Remember, no medicine can substitute for a healthy lifestyle, one that incorporates a heart-healthy diet and regular physical exercise into daily life.

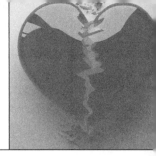

Chapter 10

Catheter-Based Therapy for Heart Disease

In 1977, a Swiss cardiologist named Andreas Gruentzig blew up a balloon-tipped catheter in a human coronary artery to clear a blockage. Overnight, he revolutionized the practice of cardiology. Up until that point, bypass surgery was the only alternative that people with unrelenting angina had to alleviate their symptoms and improve their quality of life. Before long, hundreds of thousands of patients were undergoing the procedure, called **percutaneous transluminal coronary angioplasty (PTCA)**, and another subspecialty was born: interventional cardiology. Today, the more general term **percutaneous coronary intervention (PCI)** is used to describe procedures in which many types of catheters and devices are used to improve blood flow to the heart. The term percutaneous means "through the skin" and refers to the placement of catheters into a blood vessel through a puncture in the skin.

Despite a high success rate, PTCAs were associated with complications, including abrupt closure of the artery in 7% to 8% of cases and **restenosis** (recurrence of the blockage) in

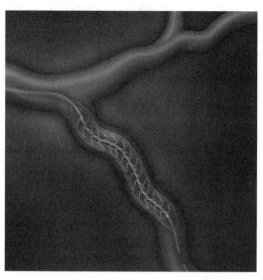

FIGURE 10.1 A stent in a human coronary artery.

about 30% of people during the first six months. In the early days of PCI, about 3% to 5% of patients required emergency bypass surgery because of complications of angioplasty.

During the 1980s and 1990s, new methods were devised to lower the incidence of abrupt closure and restenosis. In 1986, Dr. J. Puel reported on the first use of a stent in a human coronary artery (FIGURE 10.1). The introduction of stents (wire mesh devices that prevent the vessel from closing acutely) and other specialized catheters that could actually remove plaque greatly decreased the complication rate of PCIs. The need for emergency bypass surgery after PCIs in stented patients is now less than 1%. And the restenosis rate has dropped from about 30% to 18%.

Early in 2003, stents coated with medicines were introduced. The medicines used in this type of stent help prevent the overgrowth of tissue that sometimes occurs in a vessel wall that has been stented. Studies have since shown that these "drug eluting stents" (DES) markedly lower the risk of restenosis. After being in use for several years, some studies reported that the DESs had a higher risk of late clotting than so-called "bare-metal" stents. For this reason, people who have a DES inserted need to be on blood thinning medicines, usually the combination of aspirin and clopidogrel (Plavix) longer than those who receive a bare-metal stent. Current recommendations are that aspirin be continued indefinitely for both types of stents; most interventional cardiologists instruct their patients to continue clopidogrel for a minimum of one month after a bare metal stent and at least a year after a DES is used. Whether or not DESs do in fact have a higher incidence of late, in-stent clotting is still somewhat controversial.

Some other modifications of the original balloon catheters include devices that retrieve and remove clots and cutting devices that cut and remove calcified plaque from diseased coronary arteries or bypass grafts. These devices are used only in a small percentage of PCIs.

In 1985, the National Heart, Lung, and Blood Institute (NHLBI) published the results of PTCAs performed in more than 3,000 patients between 1977 and 1981. The success rate of the procedure was significantly lower in women (60%) than men (66%). In addition, women had more than double the mortality rate of men (1.8% versus 0.7%) after PTCA. In contrast, the incidence of acute myocardial infarction (MI) or emergency bypass surgery wasn't found to differ significantly between men and women. These results were confirmed in a study from the NHLBI that was published in 1993. Female gender was found to be an independent risk factor for complications of the procedure such as hemorrhage and local problems with the femoral artery. These complications, as well as the lower success rate, were thought to be due to the smaller size of arteries in women. However, women undergoing PCI also tend to be older and are more likely to be diabetic, hypertensive, and to have a history of congestive heart failure than men.

In 1997, the results from 118,548 angioplasties performed in more than 1,000 U.S. hospitals were analyzed. The report, published in the *American Journal of Cardiology* in 2001, revealed that even with stents, mortality was twice as high for women (4%) than men (2%) in patients who underwent the procedure to restore blood flow in the setting of an acute heart attack. Even in the absence of a heart attack, women who underwent stenting had about twice the mortality rate of men. This study confirmed that women who underwent either conventional PTCA or stenting had higher in-hospital mortality, whether or not they had an acute heart attack. This difference was partially explained by women's older average age and their worse cardiovascular risk profile.

Another study that looked at similar numbers of patients over the time span from 1994 to 1998 found that compared with men, women had a higher mortality rate (1.8% versus 1.0%), more strokes (0.4% versus 0.2%), and more vascular complications (5.4% versus 2.7%). However, after adjusting for clinical risk factors and body surface area (a measure of size), it was demonstrated that men and women had similar PCI mortality, although women undergoing PCI remained at a significantly higher risk of having to have repeat in-hospital procedures, stroke, and blood vessel complications. The authors of this report concluded that a person's body size, rather than gender, is an independent risk factor for mortality after PCI.

Perhaps the best news for women with regard to PCIs was published in the *Journal of the American Medical Association* in January 2002. This study looked at the results of PCI in treating acute heart attacks in a group of 1,937 people, 502 of whom were women. Despite being almost ten years older than men (the average age of the women in the study was 70.3 years versus an average age of 60.7 years for men), women had similar one-year survival rates. In fact, after age adjustment, women had a lower one-year risk of death. Given that older women have a higher incidence of complications when treated with thrombolytics (clot busters), this study confirms that whenever possible, women with acute MIs should be treated with angioplasty.

There are other, less common situations where catheter-based therapy is used. Patients with a narrowing of the mitral valve may undergo what is called **balloon valvulotomy**. In this procedure, which is performed if surgery is contraindicated, a special catheter with a balloon at the end is placed across the narrowed valve and inflated to increase the size of the mitral opening. This procedure is rarely performed nowadays. A similar procedure can be done on a narrowed aortic valve, usually in people who are so ill that it is feared they would not survive open heart surgery.

As mentioned in Chapter 6, a device delivered by catheter can be used to close the congenital abnormality called atrial septal defect, which is essentially a hole between the left and right atria. This procedure is more commonly done in children, but it can also be used to close defects in adults. A similar abnormality called a *patent foramen ovale* (PFO) can also be closed this way.

A few academic medical centers are experimenting with the implantation of artificial aortic valves via a catheter technique, and with repairing leaky mitral valves by a percutaneous approach, but these remain experimental at present.

The other area in which percutaneous procedures are having a tremendous impact on cardiology is in the treatment of certain abnormal heart rhythms. Percutaneous treatment of abnormal heart rhythms is done in a special cardiac catheterization laboratory. In this procedure, specialized catheters are inserted through small punctures in blood vessels in the groin in a manner similar to an ordinary cardiac catheterization.

Some people have abnormal heart rhythms caused by extra pathways that can conduct electrical impulses between the atria and the ventricles. This condition was called Wolff-Parkinson-White Syndrome after the first physicians to describe these accessory pathways. People with this syndrome sometimes have very rapid heart rates that are difficult to control with medication. Sometimes their arrhythmias are fatal. It's now possible to localize the accessory pathway with an electrophysiologic study (EPS). After the offending tissue is localized, it is destroyed using radio-frequency waves delivered via a special catheter. Electrical energy, laser, microwaves, and freezing have also been used to destroy accessory pathways, but these other methods aren't commonly used at present. The radio-frequency energy causes the tissue at the tip of the catheter to heat up. When the temperature exceeds 122°F, cell death occurs in the tissue closest to the catheter. This is usually a painless procedure, but sometimes it can be uncomfortable. The success rate of the procedure in patients with accessory pathways is about 85% to 90% with a rate of significant complications around 2% and a mortality rate of 0.2%. In about 8% of patients, the arrhythmia recurs.

Radio-frequency **ablation** can also be used to treat tachycardias (abnormally fast heart rhythms) arising in the atria and ventricles. Unfortunately, its use in eliminating atrial fibrillation, which affects 1 to 2 million Americans, is still in the developmental stage, and it's unclear whether it will prove to be effective in the long run.

There don't appear to be any gender-related differences in rado-frequency ablation results between men and women. When successful, it often allows patients to discontinue medications and to lead their lives free from troublesome symptoms and side effects.

In summary, PCIs have allowed cardiologists to open up narrowed coronary arteries and increase blood flow to the heart without resorting to bypass surgery. PCIs have prevented many heart attacks and allowed people with angina to live more active lives. Catheter ablation of areas of the heart that are causing abnormal heart rhythms allows people with these conditions to live more normal lives and to avoid medicines that often have serious side effects. We can expect both these procedures to be further improved and refined in the years to come.

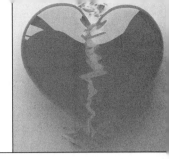

Chapter 11

Surgical Therapy for Heart Disease

Nowadays, heart surgery is so common that we tend to forget that it was unheard of throughout most of human history. When I was growing up, being a "blue baby" or having a murmur was often tantamount to a sentence of death. Historically, the first cardiac disease to be treated surgically was valvular heart disease, specifically mitral stenosis (narrowing of the valve between the left atrium and the left ventricle). As early as 1902, the possibility of treating this condition surgically was raised in the British medical journal, *Lancet*, by Sir Lauder Brunton. This possibility became a reality in 1923 when Drs. Cutler and Levine reported on the successful opening of a narrowed mitral valve in *The Boston Medical and Surgical Journal*. What makes their result astounding is that the surgery was performed on a beating heart, without the aid of the heart-lung machine, which had yet to be invented. Surgical techniques were refined over the next two decades, and by the late 1940s the operation was being performed in centers in the United States and Great Britain.

It became apparent early on that some valves were beyond repair and needed to be replaced. This was impossible before the invention of the heart-lung machine, which allowed surgeons to stop the heart while the circulation (and oxygenation) of the blood was taken over by machine. The heart-lung machine and what it does is termed **cardiopulmonary bypass (CPB)**. CPB made possible the dazzling array of cardiac operations that previous generations of cardiac specialists could only dream of. Many scientists contributed to the development of CPB during the 1940s and 1950s. The first successful operation—an atrial septal defect repair—in which a patient's circulation was totally taken over by CPB took place in 1953.

Drs. Starr and Edwards reported the first successful mitral valve replacement in 1961. Since that time, newer and better types of artificial valves have been introduced. These can be either mechanical or derived from pig or cow tissue.

Currently, the most common condition that's corrected by valve replacement surgery is calcific aortic stenosis. Although this condition is more common in men than women, the results of surgery are comparable in the two groups. Surgeons have also developed the ability to repair some leaky valves that formerly would have been replaced. In general, unlike the situation with coronary bypass surgery, the results of valve replacement or valve repair are comparable in men and women. Most centers report that operative mortality and postoperative complication rates show no gender differences for isolated heart valve surgery.

Most congenital heart disease is diagnosed and corrected in childhood. However, sometimes people, especially those with atrial septal defects, aren't diagnosed until they're adults. If their defects are too large to be closed with a catheter-based technique, their defects can be closed surgically with minimal risk.

During the 1960s, Drs. Sones and Shirey at the Cleveland Clinic developed coronary angiography, which uses x-ray dye to outline the coronary arteries. This allowed cardiologists to pinpoint the location and severity of coronary artery narrowing. In 1967 (a year before I graduated from medical school), Drs. Favaloro and Effler, also at the Cleveland Clinic, began performing operations in which they took a vein from the patient's leg and sewed one end of the vein into the aorta just above the heart and the other end into the coronary artery beyond the site where it was narrowed (FIGURE 11.1) This was the first operation that effectively increased the blood supply to the heart. Before long, tens of thousands of **coronary artery bypass graft (CABG)** surgeries were being performed each year around the globe. Today, it's by far the most common open-heart operation performed in the United States.

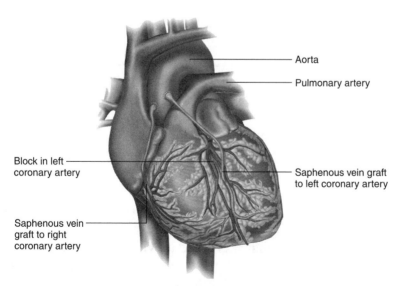

FIGURE 11.1 Coronary bypass involves using blood vessels from another part of the body to bring blood around a blocked artery in the heart.

In the early years of bypass grafting, the vast majority of people who underwent this procedure were men. The Society of Thoracic Surgeons (STS) maintains a voluntary database of patients undergoing open-heart surgery in the United States and Canada. In 1980, 83% of U.S. patients having a CABG were men and 17% were women. By 1990, the percentages were 73% men and 27% women. By 1997, the percentage of women undergoing CABG in the United States had risen only slightly to 30%. (The Canadian numbers were similar.) For 2007, the most recent year for which data are available, the STS database found that women made up 27% of the patients undergoing CABG. So even today women make up a smaller percentage of people undergoing CABG operations than would be expected, given the incidence of coronary artery disease (CAD) in older women.

The database also allowed the collection of information about the risk of dying from CABG surgery. Women have had consistently higher mortality rates than men. The 1997 death rates for CABG were 3.89% for women and 2.30% for men. This disparity had been noted since the early days of CABG surgery. The reasons are complex. As we have noted, women tend to develop CAD an average of ten to twenty years later than men do. When women undergo CABG, they tend not only to be older (by about three years on average) but are also more likely to be diabetic, hypertensive, or to have a history of heart failure. They are also more likely than men to have kidney failure and require urgent or emergency surgery. On the plus side, women undergoing CABG have had fewer prior heart attacks and have better heart function and fewer diseased arteries. The outlook for women is improving. A study in 2003 showed that although women are sicker than men both before and after CABG, they didn't have the significantly higher risk of dying from the procedure that was noted previously. Women's higher risk of complications correlated with their smaller size. Women tend to be shorter, weigh less, and thus have a smaller body surface area than men. Studies have correlated body surface area with coronary artery diameters. One study that looked at coronary artery diameters in almost 1,000 people found that the diameters of the major coronary arteries were smaller in women. More recent data about CABG results in women were compiled by researchers in Canada who reported on more than 20,000 people of whom just under 5,000 were women, who were operated on between 1991 and 2004 in British Columbia. Over that time span, thirty-day mortality dropped from 2.4% to 1.9% in men and from 5.6% to 1.9% in women.

Veins taken from the leg have traditionally been used to bypass diseased coronary arteries. A better option is to use another artery, and surgeons now have extensive experience using a chest artery called the **left internal mammary artery (LIMA)** or the radial artery in the wrist. Arterial bypasses are less likely to become diseased or blocked than veins. Unfortunately, it's more time-consuming to use arteries than veins, so they aren't used in emergency situations. At the end of one year, 95% of LIMAs are open, as opposed to 93% of vein grafts. By ten years after CABG, 83% of LIMA grafts are open; the comparable number for vein grafts is 41%. The advantage of LIMA grafts persists for up to 20 years.

Bypass surgery is about as major an operation as it's possible to have. I tell my patients that they can expect to spend about five to seven days in the hospital (assuming there are no complications) and an additional few months at home recuperating. I also tell them that it's common to be depressed after CABG surgery. Luckily, depression is almost always transient and can be treated with medication if it's unduly prolonged. Unfortunately, depression after CABG surgery is associated with an increased risk of cardiac events during the next five years. Not everyone is a candidate for this type of surgery. However, it's the procedure of choice for people with a blockage of the main left coronary artery, those with compromised function of the left ventricle, and diabetics with blockages in multiple vessels.

With the widespread use of angioplasties and stents, the population of patients undergoing CABG today is rather different from what it was in the 1970s. Today's CABG patients tend to be older and sicker. Compared to thirty years ago, they are more likely to be women and to have unstable symptoms, disease in all three major coronary arteries, or to have had prior CABG or percutaneous coronary intervention.

The possible complications of CABG include myocardial infarction, bleeding, wound infection, pneumonia, stroke, and arrhythmia. Despite these risks, we know that CABG surgery can prolong life and relieve angina symptoms. When people continue to have disabling angina despite good medical management, or if their anatomy puts them at high risk, then the potential risks of surgery are outweighed by the possible benefits. I have many patients who had surgery more than 20 years ago and are leading full, productive lives today. Now that just about all CABG patients are being treated with statins to lower their cholesterol levels, we can expect that they will do even better and live longer than people who had surgery in the pre-statin era.

Recently, there have been exciting technical advances in the field of cardiac surgery which make the procedures safer and shorten the recovery period. New devices that can stabilize the heart allow surgeons to operate without using the heart-lung machine. This avoids the potential complications that arise from the machine's use, including stroke and an increased requirement for blood transfusions. Procedures such as off-pump bypass surgery or minimally invasive cardiac surgery are particularly useful in elderly patients, who are more likely to have medical conditions such as prior stroke, kidney or lung disease, and advanced atherosclerosis, all of which increase the surgical risk. Surgeons are also using smaller chest and leg incisions, which decreases the need for narcotic pain medicine postoperatively.

~

Another way to relieve angina, called **transmyocardial revascularization with laser (TMR)**, is currently being studied in several centers. Laser energy is used to burn channels in the heart muscle after the heart has been exposed through an incision in the left chest. TMR has proven effective in relieving angina in people who aren't candidates for CABG or angioplasty. A few studies that randomized patients with refractory angina to laser therapy or medical management found that those treated with laser had more improvement in their angina, fewer cardiac events, and required fewer hospitalizations. Some studies have demonstrated improved heart performance, but this hasn't been a consistent finding. Some cardiologists feel that the laser therapy works by stimulating angiogenesis (the formation of new blood vessels), but whether or not this occurs is controversial. Others feel that the relief of angina comes about by interference with the nerves supplying the heart. Whichever is the case, it has brought relief to many people who have crippling angina and no other therapeutic options.

The first heart transplant was performed in South Africa by Dr. Christian Barnard in December 1967. Between then and March 1971, a total of 170 cardiac transplants were performed in 65 centers around the world. The early results were dismal, with 85% of heart transplant patients dying within one year. Most centers stopped performing cardiac transplants until newer treatments to combat rejection of the donated heart were developed.

Whenever foreign matter is put in the body, an immunologic response occurs. White blood cells and substances called antibodies attack the foreign tissue and destroy it. In the early 1980s, a new drug was discovered which revolutionized the field of transplant surgery. Cyclosporine selectively blocks the immune response and increases the life span of transplanted organs. By the end of the last century, more than 300 centers around the world were performing heart transplants. Currently, about 46% of heart transplants are done on people whose end-stage disease is due to CAD. Another 46% have other forms of heart muscle damage (cardiomyopathy); about 3% have valvular disease; about 2% have congenital disease (cardiac transplants have been done in infants); 2% are repeat transplants; and the rest are for miscellaneous rare conditions.

Most centers exclude people older than age 70 and those with severe disease of other organ systems, cancer, or insulin-requiring diabetes. Some exclude people who are obese. Sometimes heart assist devices are used to tide people over while they await a donor heart. All of the assist devices are associated with a significant risk of bleeding or thrombosis.

For the most part, donor hearts are obtained from otherwise healthy people who die suddenly from either a bleed into the brain, auto accident, or gunshot wound. Ideally, donor hearts are from people younger than age 55. In a survey from California conducted between the years 1995 and 1998, the average donor age was 37 years and 59.5% were male compared to 40.5% female.

The percentage of female heart transplant recipients is smaller, however. A total of 2,197 heart transplants were performed in the United States in 2000 according to the United Network for Organ Sharing. Of these, 586 (36%) were in women. The percentage of women among heart transplant recipients in 2001 was similar at 37%.

After cardiac transplantation people generally must remain on medicine to suppress the immune response for life. Multiple drugs, including cyclosporine and the steroid hormone prednisone, are used. All of these drugs have potentially serious side effects, including an increased risk of infection and certain cancers. Nevertheless, unless the donor heart is obtained from an identical twin, all heart transplant recipients need to be on immunosuppressive drugs for life.

Transplanted hearts are prone to another complication: the development of accelerated arteriosclerosis in the coronary arteries. This is found in between 20% and 50% of transplanted hearts at five years. Because the transplanted hearts have no nerve supply, people often don't experience angina pectoris when they do develop blockages. Despite this, the survival of cardiac transplant patients was 85%, 68%, and 46% at one, five, and ten years at one of the busiest transplant centers, Stanford, during the time span from 1988 to 1998. This is remarkable considering all of these patients were suffering from end-stage heart disease and had a life expectancy of a few months at the time they were transplanted.

Pacemakers and **automatic implantable cardiac defibrillators (AICDs)** require surgery for implantation, so although they are strictly speaking catheter-based (or to be really specific, wire-based) therapies, I have included them in this chapter. Because these devices have become smaller and smaller, the surgery required to implant them has become simpler. Nowadays, pacemakers and AICDs are often placed by specially trained cardiologists rather than cardiothoracic surgeons as was the case just a few years ago. The first successful human pacemakers were developed and inserted in the 1950s. The first AICD was implanted in 1979.

Pacemakers and AICDs have two parts. One part is a battery-powered generator that's inserted below the skin, usually on the upper chest. The second part consists of wires that are inserted through the vein under the collar bone and then advanced into the right atrium and right ventricle (FIGURE **11.2**). In both devices the wires are programmed to deliver a small amount of electricity to the heart, stimulating it to contract (in the case of a pacemaker) or to abort an episode of abnormal heart rhythm (in the case of AICDs).

The implantation procedures are performed under local anesthesia with sedation. An x-ray machine helps ensure that the pacing or defibrillator wires get to their correct destinations.

Pacemakers prevent the heart's rate from becoming dangerously low. They have a sensing function that allows the pacemaker to stimulate the heart when it senses that the heart rate has dropped below a certain predetermined level. Some pacemakers can also sense when the patient is exercising

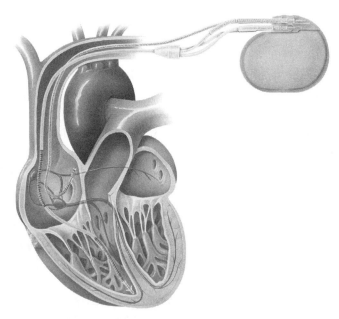

FIGURE 11.2 This device, an AICD, can sense abnormal heart rhythms and deliver an electric impulse that shocks the heart back into a normal rhythm. (Copyright 2003 Guidant Corporation.)

and increase their rate accordingly. There are people who alternate between heart rates that are too rapid (tachycardia) and heart rates that are too slow (bradycardia). A pacemaker allows the physician to give medicines to slow the tachycardia without worrying that the drugs will exacerbate the bradycardia.

Ventricular fibrillation (VF) is a common cause of **sudden cardiac death (SCD)**. It's the cause of most of the more than 350,000 SCDs that occur in the United States each year. The heart is bombarded by chaotic, extremely rapid electrical impulses and loses its ability to contract in a coordinated fashion. It quivers rather than contracts. VF can occur in the setting of an acute heart attack or can occur in people with no known heart disease. When, on rare occasions, young athletes die after blunt trauma to the chest (for example, being hit with a baseball), the cause is VF induced by a blow over the heart delivered during a vulnerable time of the cardiac cycle. There are also familial conditions that predispose people to this often fatal arrhythmia. Certain drugs are implicated in VF, notoriously cocaine. And people with severely impaired heart function are at high risk for this arrhythmia. If the heart isn't shocked back into a normal rhythm within four or five minutes, VF is always fatal.

AICDs can sense when the heart rate goes above a certain limit and can then deliver a small jolt of electricity that usually restores a normal rhythm. Multiple studies of AICDs have now demonstrated their superiority over medications in improving survival in patients at high risk of VF. In people with coronary heart disease and severe impairment of the heart's pump function, those treated with an AICD lived longer than those treated with medicine to stabilize their heart rhythm. Dr. Douglas Zipes, who participated in one of these studies, remarked that "The implantable cardiac defibrillator is like having an emergency room implanted in your chest."

Most AICDs can also perform the functions of a pacemaker. Both AICDs and pacemakers can malfunction if exposed to certain forms of electromagnetic energy. Metal detectors at airports may set off an alarm when patients with these devices walk through them. If you have a pacemaker or AICD, don't allow anyone to wave a hand-held metal detector wand near the generator/battery pack because this may cause a temporary malfunction. Microwave ovens are usually well enough insulated that they aren't a cause for concern, but other potential sources of interference include arc welders, electronic anti-theft systems, large magnets (which means you won't be able to have a diagnostic test called a magnetic resonance imaging [MRI]), and CB or ham radio antennas. When using a cellular phone, patients with these devices should hold the phone on the side opposite the battery pack. When these devices are implanted, patients are given identification cards with information about the device; these should be presented at airports or any other facility where metal detectors are in use.

There is another relatively new, exciting use for pacemakers, which proved to be a boon to a patient of mine named Sal. A big burly man in his fifties, Sal developed a cardiomyopathy about twelve years ago. He went from being very active physically to having trouble breathing if he tied his shoes. He was unable to work, which he found very depressing. His echocardiogram showed that his left ventricle was very weak. I referred him for this new type of pacing, called biventricular pacing or cardiac resynchronization therapy (CRT) and within hours after the pacemaker was inserted he said he felt "like a new man." He could exercise without getting short of breath and his echocardiogram a few months after his pacemaker was inserted showed that he now had a left ventricle that pumped normally.

Many studies have shown that pacing both the right and left ventricles can improve the function of a failing heart in selected patients with cardiomyopathy. CRT has revolution-ized our treatment of heart failure in patients who meet cri-teria for its use. Only your cardiologist can determine if you might benefit from CRT.

We can follow the progress of a failing heart by measur-ing something called the ejection fraction. This is the fraction of blood that the left ventricle pumps out to the body with each beat. We can derive this information from an echocar-diogram, a nuclear scan, a left ventricular angiogram, or a cardiac MRI study. Normally, the ejection fraction is 55% or more. When the heart muscle function begins to fail, the ejec-tion fraction falls and heart failure occurs because the organs of the body aren't getting the blood supply they need. Sal's ejection fraction went from 20% to 55% with a biventricu-lar pacemaker. Two medical device companies, Medtronic and Guidant, make biventricular pacemakers that have won approval from the Food and Drug Administration. If you suffer from severe heart failure don't be afraid to ask your physician if you might benefit from one of these devices.

In summary, cardiac surgery has saved lives and improved the quality of life for hundreds of thousands of people. Over the last five decades, open-heart surgery has gone from being a rare, highly risky undertaking to one that's used to treat heart disease in people ranging in age from newborn to ninety-plus years. Women have had a higher operative mor-tality (death within 30 days of operation) than men in most surveys of CABG. Some investigators feel that female gender itself is a risk factor for poor operative outcomes, whereas others argue that women's greater age, higher incidence of diabetes and hypertension, and smaller body surface area are the cause. However, such concerns about differences in out-come shouldn't lead to delayed treatment of women because men and women have similar long-term outcomes.

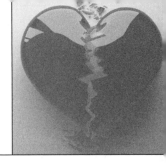

Chapter 12

Gender Bias in Medicine: Fact or Fiction?

If you really want to irk a group of male physicians, imply that there's gender bias in medicine. They will protest (vehemently) that they render the same care to women as they do to men. If you consult the medical literature you'll find articles that come down on both sides of the issue, some finding that there is indeed gender bias in medicine and others finding the opposite. I will be upfront about my own bias. *I believe that there is gender bias in medicine,* that it's pervasive, and that although it's less common than it was in the last millennium, it's still with us. Let's examine some of the data.

When I enrolled in medical school in 1964, women made up 8.9% of medical students in the United States. My premedical advisor at Barnard College told me that I would have to have better grades than most of the male applicants in order to be accepted and that I would have to convince the admissions committees of the schools to which I applied that I wouldn't "drop out" at some point in my career to have children and raise a family. Five years later, the percentage of women medical students (9.1%) hadn't changed significantly. A decade after I matriculated, women made up 22.4% of new entrants to medical schools.

What happened in the interim was the burgeoning of the women's movement. Feminist agitation brought about profound changes in the roles of women. The Supreme Court struck down anti-abortion laws in 1973, giving women greater control over their reproductive lives. Scores of books laid out the culture-wide and largely unexamined bias against women in almost all facets of life. As more and more women entered previously "male" professions, they began to campaign for change. In medicine, women demanded that they be included in clinical trials.

In cardiology, women had been systematically excluded as subjects in studies to determine the effect of various drugs on the incidence of cardiac events. Cardiovascular disease (CVD) was identified as a "male" problem and researchers assumed that results from men could be applied to women. It wasn't until 1986 that the National Institutes of Health encouraged the inclusion of women in clinical studies. Seven years later, when little progress had been made, Congress passed a law mandating the inclusion of women as subjects in clinical trials.

Since that time, women have been included in most of the large clinical trials of cardiac medicines or procedures. However, the numbers of women in these trials isn't commensurate with the numbers of women with CVD. Of eight major trials of heart failure medications involving 17,758 patients, 17% of the patients were women. Of nineteen trials of cholesterol-lowering medicines involving 46,240 patients, 19% were women. Of the 176 trials of clot busters involving 259,179 patients, 24% were women. Bear in mind that in the year 2000, 53.5% of all deaths from CVD occurred in women (46.5% occurred in men) and you'll begin to understand just how badly underrepresented women are in clinical trials. (The good news is that the number of CVD deaths in women has started to decrease. There were fewer CVD deaths in women each year between 2000 and 2004. For coronary heart disease, the death rate among women dropped from 90.1 per 100,000 in 2000 to 72.6 per 100,000 in 2004 according to the National Heart Lung and Blood Institute.)

If we examine the treatment that women receive when they present with cardiac disease or are suspected of having cardiac disease, we also find stark differences between men and women. In 1987 researchers at Albert Einstein College of Medicine in New York City published the results of a study that looked at 390 consecutive patients who had nuclear stress tests. The stress tests were done in 1982 and 1983. The researchers found that 40% of the men who had abnormal stress tests were referred for coronary angiography to determine if they should undergo bypass surgery. Only 4% of the women with abnormal tests were referred for angiography. They also found that this 10:1 ratio was independent of age. The authors did some fancy statistics on their data and concluded that "the sex differential in decisions to refer patients for cardiac catheterization cannot be explained entirely by differences in the sensitivity of tests or the rates of coronary artery disease...These findings raise the question of whether coronary artery bypass surgery is being underused in women."

A larger study published in 1991 looked at hospital data on 49,623 patient discharges in Massachusetts and 33,159 in Maryland. The study examined records on people hospitalized with coronary heart disease in 1987. The authors found that the odds of undergoing coronary angiography were 28% and 15% higher for men than women in the two states respectively. The odds of undergoing either bypass surgery or percutaneous coronary angioplasty were 45% and 27% higher for men than for women. The authors concluded that women who are hospitalized with coronary heart disease undergo fewer "major diagnostic and therapeutic procedures than men." Similar findings were reported by multiple other studies in the 1990s.

The National Registry of Myocardial Infarction is an observational database with input from more than 1,200 U.S. hospitals. Each participating hospital submits data from every patient with an acute myocardial infarction (AMI). More than 350,000 patients had AMIs between September 1990 and September 1994. The data on these patients were analyzed and published in the Archives of Internal Medicine in 1998. The authors found that in comparison with men, women were older (average age for women was 72.4 versus 65.8 for men), had a higher mortality rate even when controlled for age, and were more likely to suffer cardiac rupture whether or not they were treated with clot-dissolving medicine. When these medicines were used in women, they were treated an average of 14 minutes later than men, and women were more likely to experience major bleeding as a complication. Women were treated less frequently with aspirin, blood thinners, or beta-blockers than men. Cardiac catheterization, bypass surgery, and angioplasty were used less often in women. The authors concluded that less frequent use of clot-dissolving medicine, cardiac catheterization, bypass surgery, angioplasty, aspirin, blood thinners, and beta-blockers in women might explain, at least in part, their higher mortality rate compared with men.

Gender bias has also been found in the application of one of the newest treatments, the use of radiofrequency ablation to cure certain abnormal heart rhythms. Catheter ablation is the treatment of choice for certain specific arrhythmias called supraventricular tachycardias. An article in the *Journal of the American College of Cardiology* in 2003 found that women were referred for this procedure much later than men. There were 894 consecutive patients referred for catheter ablation in this study, 418 men and 476 women. The women had been treated for an average of 28 months longer than men after the onset of their symptoms, and were given significantly more drugs before referral. They also had more severe symptoms than men.

Multiple studies have shown that there is no difference between men and women in the success or complication rate of this procedure. The authors noted that previous reports suggest that symptoms of tachycardia are more likely to be attributed to panic, anxiety, or stress in women than in men, and that this might be delaying the diagnosis.

A hallmark study published in the prestigious *New England Journal of Medicine* in 1999 undertook to determine if physician bias contributed to the disparities in referral patterns for men and women with coronary artery disease (CAD). Physicians attending annual meetings of either the American College of Physicians in 1997 or the American Academy of Family Practice in 1996 were invited to participate in a study of clinical decision-making. Seven hundred and twenty primary care physicians, of whom 31% were women, took part. Eight actors representing each of several possible combinations of age (55 or 70 years), sex, race (black or white), level of coronary risk (low or high), and other clinical variables were recruited to portray patients in a series of standardized interviews. The physician participants viewed a recorded interview with the "patient" and were given other data. He or she then made recommendations about subsequent studies and care. The results demonstrated that the race and sex of the patient independently influenced how physicians manage chest pain. After adjusting for the probability of CAD, women were 40% less likely than men to be referred for cardiac catheterization. Black women were 60% less likely to be referred for catheterization than white men. (The data weren't analyzed separately for male and female physicians to see if there were differences based on the sex of the physician.) Yet we know from census data and various national surveys that black women younger than age 55 have more than twice the mortality rate from CAD than white women of the same age. With 11.3 deaths per 100,000, young black women have higher death rates than men younger than 45 years of age (9.2 deaths per 100,000 for black men and 5.9 deaths per 100,000 for white men). Black women between the ages of 55 and 64 are two times more likely to have a heart attack than white women. Across the board, the age-adjusted rate of CVD for black women is 72% higher than that of white women.

Another study that looked at sex and racial disparities found differences in the rates of electrocardiogram (EKG) use in patients coming to the hospital with chest pain. The American College of Cardiology and the American Heart Association recommend that all people who come to emergency departments (EDs) complaining of chest pain be given an EKG regardless of age or sex. But the National Hospital Ambulatory Medical Care Survey found spotty compliance with this recommendation when it looked at 3,356 people who came to EDs with chest pain between 1995 and 1998. People were excluded if their visit was due to injury or if they died in the ED. There were 1,664 men in the sample and 1,702 women. 2,891 (84%) of the patients had EKGs. Men were significantly more likely to have EKGs than women (86% versus 82%) and whites were significantly more likely than blacks to have EKGs (85% versus 80%). Among people younger than age 55, women and blacks were less likely to have an EKG than men, with black women being the least likely. In patients older than 55 years of age, there were no significant differences in EKG rates by sex or race.

Even the landmark Heart and Estrogen/Progestin Replacement Study (HERS) found differences in medical care and outcomes of black women compared with white women. There were 218 black women among the 2,763 study participants. All of the HERS subjects had diagnosed CVD, but the study found that black women were twice as likely to have a cardiac event as white women. Despite this, black women were less likely than white women to be treated with aspirin or the statin cholesterol-lowering medications. Black women were more likely to have high blood pressure but were less likely to have their blood pressure controlled. In addition, black women were more likely to have high levels of LDL cholesterol but were less likely than white women to be at target (LDL cholesterol less than 100 mg/dl) for this risk factor. The authors concluded: "Interventions to improve appropriate therapy and risk factor control in all women, especially black women, are needed."

One study that did look at physician gender and its impact on sex differences in cardiac catheterization found that women who had a myocardial infarction were referred for catheterization less often than men whether they were treated by a male or female physician. More than 100,000 patients were involved in this study, which looked at hospital admissions in Medicare patients between January 1994 and February 1995. Even after adjustments for baseline differences, men treated by male physicians were most likely to undergo cardiac catheterization and women treated by female physicians were least likely. Women had fewer catheterizations than men did whether treated by male physicians (38.6% women versus 50.8% men) or female physicians (34.8% women versus 45.8% men). The authors concluded "sexual discrimination, principally by male physicians towards women, does not explain sex-associated disparities in cardiac catheterization use after an acute myocardial infarction. However, other attitudes common to both male and female physicians may contribute to lower rates of cardiac procedure use in women."

One such attitude is that male and female doctors tend to see women as more emotional and therefore more likely to have a psychologic cause for their symptoms. In a study at the State University of New York, male and female medical students were given case reports of a 48-year-old man and a 58-year-old woman with equal risks of heart disease. The patients had identical symptoms and half of them were said to be experiencing job stress. The addition of the job stress factor brought out striking gender bias in diagnosis and referral. By and large, male and female medical students referred the anxious male patient to a cardiologist whereas most of the students sent the anxious female patient with the same symptoms to a psychologist.

Another study used an actress performing the role of a patient with cardiac symptoms during a videotaped interview. The actress used two distinct styles to portray her symptoms. In one version of the interview, the actress gave a business-like portrayal; in the other she gave a more dramatic presentation. Two groups of internists viewed the interviews. The actress used the same script in both versions of the interview. The diagnosis suspected by the physicians differed depending on the portrayal they saw. A cardiac diagnosis was suspected 50% of the time for the business-like portrayal but only 13% of the time for the more dramatic portrayal. Similarly, internists viewing the dramatic portrayal were far less likely to order further cardiac testing.

Other studies have tried to refute the thesis that there's gender bias in the treatment or evaluation of women with suspected heart disease. One study found that academic cardiologists referred women to cardiac catheterization less often than men (18% versus 27%) but that this difference was completely accounted for by the lower probability of CAD in women. Another study found that equal numbers of men and women were referred for coronary artery bypass graft surgery (CABG) after catheterization (46% of men and 44% of women) when significant CAD was found. Some physicians justify their lower referral of female patients for aggressive management by pointing out the generally worse outcomes in women. Unlike earlier studies of CABG and percutaneous coronary intervention mortality in women, the large Bypass Angioplasty Revascularization trial reported in 1998 that women with multivessel CAD undergoing revascularization had similar in-hospital mortality and better five-year survival rates than men.

If we look at the sheer numbers, it's hard not to conclude that women receive less intensive care than men. The American Heart Association in its 2002 Heart and Stroke Statistical Update noted that of the 472,000 outpatient cardiac catheterizations performed in the United States in 1996, 37% were done on women. In 1999, only 34% of 601,000 angioplasties were done on women. In 2000, 27% of 2,198 heart transplants were performed in women.

Finally, women may be slow to think that their symptoms could be due to heart disease. Various studies have shown that women having heart attacks seek medical attention about an hour later than men do. (However women aren't to blame for the fact that once they arrive in the ED they wait longer than men to receive an EKG or treatment.) Women are less likely to think that they are at risk for heart disease and therefore may ignore symptoms that would have a man rushing to the hospital. A recent study from Scotland found that women having heart attacks often called their physicians first, whereas men went straight to the ED. Women may also prefer less aggressive, invasive treatment.

I believe that with increased education of both the medical profession and women themselves, gender disparity in the diagnosis and treatment of women with heart disease will decrease dramatically, if not disappear. One of my goals in writing this book is to arm women with the knowledge they need to lower their risk of developing cardiac disease, and to recognize symptoms of heart disease when they do occur.

A clear concise history is a tremendous boon to your physician. I was taught in medical school that you can't make the correct diagnosis without taking a good history, and that you can't take a good history unless you know the diagnosis. This old saw has some truth to it but a patient who can accurately describe her symptoms will make her physician's job a lot simpler. Don't be afraid to insist on a cardiac work-up if you feel your symptoms could be coming from your heart. If you think that your symptoms are being trivialized, brushed off, or attributed to "stress" perhaps it's time to look for another physician.

How can you find a physician you can trust? My own bias is that if you have, or suspect you have, cardiac disease, you're best served by seeing a board-certified cardiologist. Such a physician has completed a three-year residency in internal medicine as well as three or four additional years of fellowship in an approved cardiology training program. During the fellowship years, trainees become proficient in performing and interpreting the various cardiac diagnostic tests and in evaluating and treating patients with the full gamut of heart conditions. The elective fourth year may be spent performing angioplasties or electrophysiologic studies or concentrating on echocardiography or nuclear medicine. After completing the fellowship, candidates for board certification must take and pass a comprehensive examination. Only then are they called "board-certified" cardiologists, with the diploma to prove it. Your local medical society will have a list of board-certified cardiologists who practice in your area. In addition, many hospitals have referral services that can direct you to board-certified specialists who practice on their staffs.

More and more hospitals are setting up specialized centers for women with heart disease. These centers are places where women can be certain that their complaints will be taken seriously by staff who are well aware of the differences in how cardiac disease may manifest in women. The Women's Cardiac Center at the Miriam Hospital, which I direct, is one such center in southern New England. And lastly, there are multiple sites on-line that can help you to locate a physician. The American Medical Association's web site is one of many that provide information on thousands of medical practices in the United States.

After you've located a potential cardiologist, there's no substitute for meeting face to face. Your insurance company may require you to have a referral from your primary care physician before it will pay for this evaluation. Be forewarned that some health maintenance organizations penalize primary care physicians financially if they refer more than a specified number of patients to a specialist. Be assertive and insist on being referred. Before your first appointment, organize your medical history so that you can give a clear, concise account of your symptoms and provide pertinent family or social history. ALWAYS be honest in answering your physician's questions. He or she is bound by confidentiality laws to keep anything you relate strictly between the two of you unless you give permission for the information to be shared with other health professionals. (Obviously, this doesn't apply to situations where another's life will be put in danger if the information isn't divulged. For example, if you tell your physician you've decided to purchase a gun and take out your boss, expect a visit from the police.)

Most people can tell from the get-go if they feel comfortable with a physician. One who seems rushed, indifferent, or condescending is one to be avoided. Look for a cardiologist who takes the time to obtain a complete history, perform a thorough physical examination, and explain in detail what tests and drugs are needed and why. This is the person you will be entrusting your heart to. Be sure he or she is worthy of that honor.

Remember that there's no substitute for a trusted and caring physician. You and your physician must form a therapeutic alliance. *You* must strive to maximize your healthy behaviors and your physician must treat those risk factors that detract from your health. Sometimes when I tell patients that they have to make radical lifestyle changes (such as giving up a two–pack–a–day smoking habit) they say: "But doc, we all have to die sometime." My response is: "That is true. The trick is to stay healthy until the second you go." Death is inevitable, but decades of suffering and crippling symptoms before the terminal event aren't. In many ways, how you spend the last years of life is up to you.

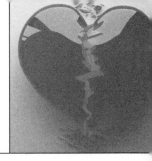

Chapter 13

What's on the Horizon?
New and Emerging Treatments

During the last four decades our ability to cure and treat heart disease has increased exponentially. We can modify risk factors with ever more effective medications, and we can correct structural heart problems with ever more sophisticated surgical operations and devices. These advances were made possible by the knowledge gained from scientific study. The explosion of medical knowledge over the last half of the twentieth century and the first decade of the twenty-first century has been without parallel in human history. We can expect this march of progress to continue. In this chapter, I will briefly touch on some exciting developments in the field of cardiology and cardiac surgery.

A new class of medicines to treat angina has been developed in the last few years. Called potassium channel activators, they have been shown in a recent clinical trial not only to relieve angina but to reduce mortality, nonfatal heart attack, and hospitalizations for angina in patients treated with the active drug compared with those treated with placebo. The study involved patients in Europe treated with nicorandil. While not yet available in the United States, this class of medicines holds much promise.

Rather than treating the symptom, what if you could abolish the underlying process? What if you could actually grow new arteries that were free of plaque? Angiogenesis is the term used to describe the growth and proliferation of new blood vessels. Scientists have identified several growth factors that stimulate angiogenesis. These growth factors have been studied in dogs and pigs. Trials have demonstrated the safety of these growth factors in humans but we don't know the doses or best methods of delivering these agents. Also, they haven't been shown to be beneficial thus far. Additional studies are underway to answer the questions about dosage and delivery and to determine if new, functional blood vessels can be formed.

What if rather than just growing new blood vessels you could grow a whole new heart? This is probably the most exciting area of new research; it involves stem cells, which have been in the news. Stem cells are cells that can divide indefinitely when grown in tissue culture and can give rise to specialized cells. Stem cells may be **totipotent** (able to give rise to any tissue or organ) or **pluripotent** (able to give rise to most tissues or organs). For example, a fertilized egg is totipotent. In humans, about four days after fertilization and several cycles of cell division, the totipotent cells begin to specialize forming a structure called the blastocyst. The outer layer of the blastocyst becomes the placenta and the inner layer becomes the embryo. The cells in the inner cell layer are pluripotent; they can give rise to most (but not all) types of cells. At present, human pluripotent stem cells are derived from embryos left over from in vitro fertilization procedures or from fetal tissue obtained from terminated pregnancies.

Using stem cells from these sources is controversial because of the opposition of those whose religious beliefs prohibit abortion. (In August 2001, President Bush announced guidelines for stem cell use. He said that federally-funded researchers could use embryonic stem cells already produced anywhere in the world but couldn't themselves destroy embryos and couldn't use cells produced after his proclamation. He noted that as a result of private research, several dozen stem cell lines already existed. He said that using these cell lines for study was permissible. Privately funded researchers are free to use embryonic stem cells from any source.)

After further specialization, pluripotent stem cells lose some of their capacity; they become **multipotent** stem cells that give rise to cells with a specific function. Two examples are bone marrow stem cells that give rise to the various types of blood cells and skin stem cells that give rise to the various types of skin cells. Bone marrow stem cells continually replenish our supply of blood cells. Skin stem cells perform the same function for skin, which we shed continuously. Both are necessary for life and are found in adults as well as embryos and children. Unfortunately, multipotent stem cells haven't been found in all types of adult tissue. (We haven't isolated a human cardiac stem cell.) Research continues, however, and discoveries in this area are increasing.

What we're learning from studies in animals and humans is that multipotent stem cells can, under certain conditions, grow into cells of a different organ than would be expected given the cells' origin. For example, studies in mice and humans have shown that bone marrow stem cells can differentiate into liver cells. More pertinent to the heart, another study using mice has demonstrated the ability of bone marrow stem cells to become cardiac muscle cells. The mice had myocardial infarctions caused by tying off a coronary artery. Bone marrow cells were then injected into the contracting heart muscle at the borders of the damaged tissue. Nine days later the investigators found that newly formed heart muscle cells derived from the bone marrow cells formed 68% of the damaged portion of the heart. These cells differentiated not only into myocardial muscle cells, but also into blood vessel lining cells and smooth muscle cells. In comparison with the control mice, which hadn't received the bone marrow cells, the treated mice had smaller heart attacks and better cardiac function. No such study has been done to date in humans. We don't yet know if bone marrow stem cells can differentiate into cardiac cells in humans. However, researchers in France have reported promising results using stem cells taken from a man's thigh muscle. They described the case of a 72-year-old man who had a heart attack. Physicians transplanted stem cells from his thigh and found at autopsy 18 months later that the cells had survived and evolved into a well-developed, functioning part of the heart muscle.

Adult stem cells have significant limitations. Besides not being found for all cell and tissue types, they typically occur in minute quantities, are difficult to isolate and purify, and may decrease in number with age. They may contain more genetic mutations because their DNA has been exposed over a lifetime to harmful substances such as drugs or tobacco. To obtain stem cells, it may be necessary to perform more-than-trivial invasive procedures. For example, the only way to obtain nerve stem cells to treat epilepsy is to remove a portion of the brain, which isn't a minor undertaking. Despite such limitations, research on adult stem cells is supported with federal funds and will continue.

We're a long way from growing new hearts from stem cells, but research on all types of stem cells will continue and will allow us to unlock the mysteries of human development. The study of stem cells will help us to learn how cells specialize, to better understand cell division, and to identify the genes that control these processes. It isn't farfetched to believe that this knowledge will allow us to cure or prevent atherosclerosis, cancer, and birth defects, to name but a few of the scourges that still exact a staggering toll.

In the field of cardiac surgery, an emerging advance is the use of "beating heart surgery." In these procedures, patients do not have to be put on the heart-lung machine in order to bypass diseased arteries. Robotic techniques are being developed which will lessen the morbidity and mortality associated with many cardiac surgeries. The daVinci robot, the most widely used system in the United States, is currently being used in bypass operations and procedures to abolish atrial fibrillation, close atrial septal defects, and repair mitral valves.

New devices to assist failing hearts are being developed and improved upon. These often serve as a "bridge to transplantation" allowing critically ill patients to survive until a donor heart becomes available. Devices like pacemakers and AICDs will no doubt undergo improvements in their capabilities and continued decrease in their size. Research is ongoing to lessen the risk of restenosis in arteries that have been stented, and lower the risk of late clotting.

With the mapping of the human genome, our understanding of the genetic basis of disease is growing by leaps and bounds. Genetic research will make it possible to better predict which patients will respond to which medications and gene therapy may someday cure or prevent hereditary cardiac diseases such as inherited cardiomyopathies, or lipid disorders like familial hypercholesterolemia.

The twentieth century saw astounding advances in medical science. It's likely that scientists of the twenty-first century will surpass those achievements, allowing us to extend healthy human life to undreamed of limits.

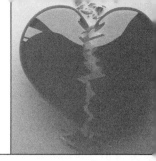

Chapter 14

A Look Back at the History of Medicine (We've Come a Long Way, Baby!)

There is nothing in this chapter you need to know to maintain a healthy heart, but if humility is the beginning of wisdom, I hope you'll be humbled, as I have been, to learn of the immense strides that have been made in the healing arts, from their first glimmerings to the miracles we take for granted today. Many books have been written about the history of medicine. This chapter leaves out many who made important contributions, but I have tried to hit the high points in the long saga that comprises the march of medical progress.

The earliest surviving writings on medicine appeared about five thousand years ago. In China, around 3000 B.C., the emperor Shen Nung set forth his knowledge of a large number of drugs and poisons (including opium, arsenic, and iron) in the *Pen Tsao* or *The Great Herbal*. A few hundred years later the *Nei Ching* or *The Book of Medicine* appeared. Believed to be the work of Hwang Ti, it contains the earliest known description of the circulation of the blood: "All the blood in the body is under the control of the heart...The blood current flows continuously in a circle and never stops." (Unfortunately, this knowledge never made it to the West. It would take more than four millennia before the circulation of the blood was described again by a British physician.)

During the same era, a man named Sekhet'enanach was physician to one of the Egyptian pharaohs who lived about 3000 B.C. He treated a condition of the king's nose and was rewarded with a self-portrait fashioned in stone. A generation or so later, Imhotep was grand vizier to the Pharaoh Zoser. A noted politician and architect, Imhotep was also worshipped for many centuries after his death as the god of Medicine.

The Code of Hammurabi, the oldest surviving collection of laws, was drawn up by one of the earliest kings of Babylon. Hammurabi ruled from about 1948 to 1905 B.C. and had his edicts engraved on a pillar of stone. The Code contains the earliest reference to laws regulating the practice of medicine. It stated, "If the doctor shall treat a gentleman and shall open an abscess with a bronze knife and shall preserve the eye of the patient, he shall receive ten shekels of silver...if the doctor shall kill the patient...his hands shall be cut off." From this we can deduce that at this early date, physicians were men and bad outcomes were devoutly to be avoided.

In the Old Testament, the only operation that's mentioned is circumcision, and this was performed by a priest, or mohel, as it is to this day. Although it has little in the way of references to medicines, the Bible does contain many injunctions on personal and community hygiene, making the Jews the earliest people to demonstrate a concern for public health.

The origins of the scientific medicine we practice today date back to Hippocrates, who was born on the Greek island of Kos in 460 B.C. Hippocrates was said to be a descendant of the god Aesculapius, who received instruction from Chiron, a centaur who was worshipped as the god of surgery. Chiron, in turn, received instruction in the healing arts from Apollo, the god of Health. This fanciful genealogy aside, in Hippocrates we see for the first time an attempt to separate medicine from magic, to record systematic observations of patients, and to set high standards for those who wished to follow what he called "The Art."

When I graduated from medical school in 1968, I recited the Hippocratic Oath, as have legions of other physicians over the centuries. Although parts of it are outmoded (Hippocrates cautioned physicians from using surgery to remove stones), its core principles of helping the sick, abstaining from intentionally causing harm, maintaining confidentiality, and honoring our teachers remain as valid today as they did in ancient Greece. In other writings, Hippocrates urged physicians "not to be too grasping, but to consider carefully your patient's means. Sometimes give your services for nothing." Lacking a stethoscope, he listened to the chest with his ear and described abnormal sounds in disease states. He wrote that diseases arose from external factors, not from divine or sacred causes (as most ancient people believed) and noted the effect of food, occupation, and climate on illness. He also urged healers to practice the art of forecasting: "He will carry out treatment best if he knows beforehand from the present symptoms what will take place later on." Hippocrates was fond of simple remedies, such as honey and vinegar, but was also a good surgeon. In advice that's still adhered to today he instructed surgeons: "The nails neither to exceed nor come short of the finger tips...Practice all the operations with each hand and with both together." He gave details for the use of boiled water and emphasized the need for "ability, speed, and painlessness."

With the rise of the Roman Empire many Greek physicians found their way to Rome—some as slaves, others as traveling healers. Marcus Porcius Cato (called "the Censor"), who included Greeks among his many pet peeves (public displays of affection was another; he had Manlius expelled from the Roman senate for kissing his wife in public), wrote to his son: "The Greeks are an intractable and iniquitous race. They have sworn to kill all barbarians with their drugs and they call us barbarians. Remember that I forbid physicians for you."

Pliny the Elder, who died in the eruption of Vesuvius that destroyed Pompeii and Herculaneum in 79 A.D., wrote "It is unfortunate that there is no law to punish ignorant physicians, and that capital punishment is never inflicted on them. Yet they learn by our suffering and they experiment by putting us to death." The poet Martial seemed to envision a modern teaching hospital when one of his epigrams noted:

I'm ill. I send for Symmachus; he's here
A hundred students following in the rear;
All paw my chest, with hands as cold as snow.
I had no fever but I have it now.

Despite this carping, medicine was advancing in public esteem. And for the first time history records the presence of women in the healing profession. Women physicians practiced in ancient Rome. Some of them wrote abortion manuals, which were popular among aristocratic ladies and prostitutes. One woman physician, Metrodora, wrote a treatise on diseases of the womb that still exists. Julius Caesar enfranchised the profession of medicine in Rome, and the first emperor, his grandnephew Augustus, exempted it from taxation. Celsus, a member of the noble Cornelius family, wrote an encyclopedia of which only the eight books dealing with medicine survive. In the third book he lists four cardinal signs of inflammation that are still taught today: *calor* (heat), *rubor* (redness), *tumor* (swelling), and *dolor* (pain). He describes venereal disease, gout, jaundice, palsy, and hydrocephalus. He discusses blood-letting, operations for goiter, hernia, stone removal, tonsillec-tomy, and the treatment of wounds. He lists drugs and their uses including mandrake, poppy, and myrrh.

The most famous practitioner of medicine in the Roman era was Galen. He was born in the second century A.D. in what is now Turkey. He began the study of medicine at the age of seventeen and attended schools in Palestine, Greece, Cyprus, Crete, and Alexandria. He served as a surgeon at a gladiator's school in Asia Minor and practiced in Rome from 164 to 168 A.D. Galen was noted for telling the truth, even if it was unpalatable. His honesty in exposing the ignorance of some of his medical colleagues in Rome provoked their anger and caused him to have to flee for his life. In 169, how-ever, he was recalled to Rome by the emperor Marcus Aure-lius to care for his son Commodus. Galen remained there until his death thirty years later. He wrote extensively, cor-responded with patients from every province, and compiled 500 volumes of which 118 survived the depredations of the Dark Ages. Roman law forbade the dissection of humans, but Galen made many contributions to the study of anatomy. He dissected animals, including Barbary apes, and trans-ferred the knowledge gained there to humans. He showed that the excised heart could beat for a time outside the body and proved that arteries contain not air, as had been thought up till then, but blood. He described the mechanics of respi-ration and conjectured that the most important element in the air was the one that was active in combustion. He showed that each side of the brain controls motion on the opposite side of the body and described the spinal cord and nerves.

Galen was hardly without error. He took up Hippocrates' belief in the four humors—blood and phlegm, black and yel-low bile—and their influence on disease states. He ridiculed those practitioners who used spells and magic but accepted divination by dreams and believed in the influence of the moon on the condition of patients. (In fairness to Galen, most physicians who work nights in emergency departments dread full moons, convinced that "the crazies come out" on those nights more than on any other night.) His errors, particularly those in anatomy (he taught that the blood was formed in the liver and that the blood vessels arose there, not in the heart), were perpetuated for centuries. Most of his writings were lost in the chaos of the barbarian invasions, but some were preserved by Arab scholars and were translated back from Arabic into Latin from the eleventh century on. He was revered by practitioners of medieval medicine. Those who questioned his teachings were regarded as medical heretics.

Wracked by barbarian invasions, the Roman Empire fell in the fifth century A.D. and Europe entered the Dark Ages. Two very different institutions kept alive the knowledge gleaned by the ancients. In Europe, monasteries were founded and men flocked to them despite the required vows of poverty, chastity, and obedience. Monasteries provided a haven from the political instability and constant warfare of the time. Monks tilled the soil but more importantly they toiled for years copying and translating the authors of classic antiquity. Unfortunately, the Church also retarded the march of medical knowledge by its emphasis on sin and its denigration of the body. In the teachings of the Church, disease was regarded as punishment for sin and prayer, fasting, and repentance were the preferred treatments. Unfortunately, not all Christians revered secular knowledge. In A.D. 391, a mob of Christian fanatics set fire to the greatest library of ancient times in Alexandria, Egypt, destroying many priceless works of learning.

The second group that preserved and expanded medical knowledge before the Renaissance consisted of the followers of Islam. Founded by the prophet Mohammed in the seventh century A.D., Islam was tolerant and respectful of learning in its inception. Mohammed wrote of medicine: "O servant of God, use medicine, because God hath not created a pain without a remedy for it." Not content to just copy Greek texts, Muslim physicians added much to the store of medical knowledge by their observations and experiments. The words alcohol, syrup, sugar, and alkali, among many others, are derived from Arabic. Hospitals were established throughout the lands where Islam held sway, and medical students trained within these institutions. A tenth century Persian physician, Rhazes, was the first to differentiate between smallpox and measles. He was also the first to use animal gut in sutures. Not without a sense of humor, his written works included *On the Fact That Even Skillful Physicians Cannot Cure All Diseases* and *Why Ignorant Physicians, Laymen, and Women Have More Success than Learned Medical Men.*

The most famous practitioner of Arabian medicine was Avicenna, who lived from A.D. 908 to 1037. A Persian, like Rhazes, he was a child prodigy who memorized the Koran before the age of ten. He was appointed as a court physician at age eighteen. He wrote a landmark text, the *Canon of Medicine* in which he incorporated the teachings of Galen and the philosopher Aristotle. His textbook was used in medical schools in Europe as late as 1650. Avicenna was the first to recognize that tuberculosis was a contagious disease and he wrote treatises on the reduction of fractures, the importance of clean water, the care of the aged, and the therapeutic value of music.

In the twelfth century, Maimonides, a Jew who was born in Cordova, Spain when it was ruled by the Moors, became the most famous physician of his time. He traveled throughout northern Africa and the Middle East after being banished from Spain because he wouldn't convert. He acquired a reputation so outstanding that he was appointed physician to Saladin, the famous Saracen leader who fought against the Christians in the Crusades, a series of wars Christendom undertook to reclaim Jerusalem. The legendary crusader King Richard the Lion-Hearted was said to want Maimonides as his own physician, but Maimonides declined, no doubt politely. Maimonides wrote extensively. Included in his works are a guide to personal health written for Saladin's son entitled *Book of Counsel, Guide for the Perplexed*, in which he attempted to reconcile religion and medicine.

Maimonides stressed the importance of character and taught that the worst bite of all was the bite of "a fasting man." He advised simple drugs rather than complex mixtures and searched for causes of disease in the natural world rather than in magic and spells. Commenting on marital relations he wrote: "When cohabiting, neither husband nor wife should be in a state of intoxication, lethargy, or melancholy. The wife should not be asleep at the time." In contrast to the arrogance that sometimes characterized physicians he prayed: "May I never forget that the patient is a fellow creature in pain. May I never consider him merely a vessel of disease."

The earliest medical school in Europe was established at Salerno, Italy where a health resort had existed since the early days of Rome. Allegedly founded in the ninth century by a Jew, a Greek, a Christian, and an Arab, the Salerno school became famous by the eleventh century, only to be superseded in the thirteenth century by the university at Bologna. For the first time since the Roman Empire, the presence of women practitioners and teachers was recorded. Some of their names have come down to us: Constanza, Rebecca, and Trotula. Trotula authored a book on obstetrics, written about A.D. 1050. Students had to be twenty-one to begin their medical studies at Salerno. The training took five years, after which the candidates had to take and pass examinations. They were required to swear an oath to treat the poor for free, not to administer noxious drugs, and to support the school. After this, the candidate was entitled to call himself "doctor" and to practice medicine. It was here that medical practitioners were first called "doctor" from the Latin word for teacher, *doctus*. The School at Salerno accepted students without regard to religion or nationality and was the first in Europe to award a degree after a defined course of study and the passing of examinations.

The Salerno school went into decline in the thirteenth century (although it existed until 1811 when it was closed by Napoleon). The torch of medical learning was passed on to newer schools that were established in Montpellier, Paris, Padua, and Bologna. The most famous of Bologna's medical sons, Theodoric of Lucca, wrote a surgical text that revealed him to be ahead of his time. He recognized that pus wasn't an inevitable or desirable accompaniment of wound healing, as was believed, and introduced the use of alcohol as an antiseptic. He practiced a crude form of anesthesia by having patients inhale from a sponge impregnated with opium and mandragora. Another great teacher at Bologna, William of Salicet, distinguished between bleeding from arteries and veins and advocated the study of anatomy. Mondino de Luzzi published the first practical anatomy manual in 1316. He carried out human dissections assisted by his female pupil, Alexandra Galiani, and despite many errors (he described the heart as having three ventricles), his Anothomia remained a standard text for two centuries. However, medieval medicine continued many of the fallacies of the ancients; it had little to offer the vast majority of suffering patients who fell into its clutches, and surgery for the most part was practiced by barbers.

All of that was about to change with the flowering of learning and art which came to be known as the Renaissance. Beginning in Italy towards the end of the fourteenth century, the Renaissance facilitated a sea change in the thinking of men, in their relationship to religion, and in their understanding of the natural world. In 1543, two revolutionary works were published: Copernicus' *De revolutionibus orbium coelestium*, a text about the revolution of the heavenly bodies, and Vesalius' *De humani corporis fabrica*, a text about human anatomy.

Born in Brussels in 1514, Vesalius came from a long line of medical practitioners. As a child he dissected various small animals. He was educated in Louvain and Paris. He engaged in "body-snatching" expeditions and was able to obtain the bodies of executed criminals for dissection. These studies allowed Vesalius to prove that the teaching at the time was full of errors and that Galen shouldn't have been regarded as the final authority. He was only twenty-eight when his seminal work was published, and it laid the groundwork upon which Harvey in a later century was able to base his discovery of the circulation of the blood. The work included detailed and accurate drawings of anatomic figures, which served as models for generations of artists and gave medical students their first accurate instruction in the anatomy of the human body.

Vesalius was consulted by royalty. He was called to the bedside of Henry II of France who had received a lance wound to the eye in a friendly tournament with the captain of the Scottish Guard. (Henry was the father-in-law of Mary Stuart, later known as Mary, Queen of Scots, who would suffer beheading at the order of her cousin, Queen Elizabeth I of England). Also called in on that case was Ambrose Paré, but the efforts of the two most famous medical men of their time were unsuccessful and Henry died of his wound. Vesalius drowned in a shipwreck in 1564 while returning from a pilgrimage to Jerusalem.

As has so often occurred in history, war was a spur to the acquisition of scientific knowledge. The man who is considered the Father of Modern Surgery, Ambrose Paré (1510–1590) started out as a barber-surgeon but soon gave up the tonsorial side of his profession and concentrated on surgery. During his lifetime, France was engaged in wars with Germany, England, Italy, and its own Huguenots (Protestants). Paré joined the French King's army and spent thirty years as an army surgeon. He proved that wounds were better treated with a "digestive of eggs, oil of roses, and turpentine" than the boiling oil which was then standard therapy, noting that those whose wounds were dressed with the digestive had little pain, while those treated with boiling oil were "feverish, with great pain, and swelling of their wounds." He described the use of ligatures or ties rather than cautery to stem hemorrhage, ended the practice of castration in hernia operations, and invented forceps. When he was elderly he wrote *Journeys in Diverse Places*, an entertaining look at the life of a sixteenth century army surgeon. He taught that "it is always wise to hold out hope to the patient, even if the symptoms point to a fatal issue," advice that is followed by wise and compassionate physicians to this day.

The foundations of modern science were laid during the Renaissance. Learned men questioned the accepted authority of the Church and State. Blind belief was supplanted by knowledge acquired from experiments. Francis Bacon (1561–1626), a philosopher and statesman, argued that truth was derived not from authority but from experience. This argument was taken to heart by men of all the sciences, including medicine.

~

If cardiology can be said to have a beginning, it isn't far-fetched to say that it dates from the publication of William Harvey's *De Motu Cordis*, or the *Anatomical Treatise on the Movement of the Heart and Blood in Animals* in 1628. Harvey was born at Folkestone in 1578, the eldest of seven sons. He was educated at Cambridge and Padua. He graduated with high honors as Doctor of Medicine in 1602. He returned to England where he practiced in London and within a few years became a Fellow of the College of Physicians and an attending doctor at St. Bartholomew's Hospital (which remains a noted teaching hospital to this day). Harvey dedicated his landmark work to his sovereign, Charles I of England, noting that: "the knowledge of his own Heart cannot be unprofitable to a King."

Before Harvey's discovery, it was thought that the blood moved in a to and fro motion and that it passed from the right to the left side of the heart through pores in the septum dividing the two ventricles. Harvey conducted experiments on both warm- and cold-blooded animals. He proved that the heart is a muscular pump whose action gives rise to the pulse. He tied off arteries and veins and by dint of careful observation was able to arrive at his belief that "there might...be a motion, as it were, in a circle." His work was greeted with cries of outrage by the leading physicians of the day, but his reasoned response to their criticisms won him more supporters and he lived to see his views widely accepted. Not content to rest on these laurels, he also published the first original work in English on obstetrics.

Four other British scientists of this era also made significant contributions to knowledge. Robert Boyle (1627–1691) showed that air was necessary to life. He created a vacuum with an air pump and showed that in a vacuum a candle couldn't burn and small animals died. If he reintroduced air within a short time, the animals recovered. His assistant, Robert Hooke, a microscopist who first used the word "cell," was also the first person to demonstrate the use of artificial respiration, which he performed by blowing into the windpipe of an animal.

Two Cornishmen, Richard Lower and John Mayow, demonstrated that the entrance of air into the blood was necessary for the maintenance of life. Mayow wrote: "some constituent of the air necessary to life enters into the blood in the act of breathing." He anticipated the discovery of oxygen by noting that it wasn't the entire air that maintained life because when a small animal was sealed up in a vessel the animal died even though the air remained.

It was during the next century that a description of that twentieth century scourge, arteriosclerotic heart disease, was first recorded. William Heberden the Elder was a graduate of Cambridge and subsequently practiced in London where he numbered King George III and Samuel Johnson among his patients. His *A Disorder of the Breast* was first read before the Royal College of Physicians in 1768 and was included in his *Commentaries*, a compendium of notes on patients and diseases culled from over forty years of practice. He had studied Latin, as did all learned men of the era, and the cardinal symptom of arteriosclerotic heart disease is known to us by the Latin term he first used to describe it, angina pectoris. After discussing other kinds of chest discomfort Heberden wrote:

> But there is a disorder of the breast marked with strong and peculiar symptoms, considerable for the kind of danger belonging to it, and not extremely rare, which deserves to be mentioned more at length. The seat of it, and sense of strangling, and anxiety with which it is attended, may make it not improperly be called angina pectoris.

They who are afflicted with it, are seized while they are walking, (more especially if it be up hill, and soon after eating) with a painful and most disagreeable sensation in the breast... but the moment they stand still, all this uneasiness vanishes... The pain is... more often inclined to the left than to the right side. It likewise very frequently extends from the breast to the middle of the left arm... Males are most liable to this disease, especially such as have past their fiftieth year.

Heberden noted the tendency for the symptoms to progress and to occur with less exertion, and: "After it has continued a year or more will not cease so instantaneously upon standing still ... " He reported that he had seen nearly one hundred patients with this disorder, of whom only three were women. He noted the frequency with which afflicted patients died suddenly. After more than two centuries, Heberden's description has hardly been bettered. Physicians still sometimes refer to the symptom caused by insufficient blood flow to the heart as "Heberden's angina."

The eighteenth century also saw the popularization of one of the earliest cardiac drugs, digitalis. William Withering (1741–1779) was a graduate of the medical school in Edinburgh. Originally from Shropshire, he knew that a popular folk remedy there for "dropsy" (swelling) was an extract of foxglove leaves, taken as a tea. He realized that dropsy could be due to cardiac disease. In 1785, he wrote in *An Account of the Foxglove* that careful use of digitalis was an effective treatment.

The nineteenth century saw the invention of the instrument that still dangles from the neck of every cardiologist. Rene Laennec was a Frenchman who studied medicine in Paris after serving an apprenticeship with his uncle who was a physician. It was already common practice for physicians to listen to patients' chests with the naked ear. However, one day Laennec was examining a patient whose obesity made it difficult to hear heart sounds. He had noted two children playing with a log of wood, one tapping on one end while the other listened at the other. Laennec rolled up paper into a cylinder and applied one end to the patient's chest and the other to his ear. He wrote that he could hear the heart "in a manner more clear and distinct than I had ever been able to do by the immediate application of the ear." He went on to fashion a stethoscope of wood and it became popular in France as well as other countries.

The nineteenth century saw an explosion of knowledge in the fields of physiology, bacteriology, and pathology all of which paved the way for the stunning medical advances of the twentieth century. Pasteur, Koch, Bernard, Muller, and Virchow were some of the scientists of this era whose contributions to knowledge are incalculable. In the field of cardiology, William Stokes published an early (perhaps the first) cardiology text, *Diseases of the Heart and Aorta*. He postulated that the state of the heart muscle was more important than the state of the cardiac valves. He, along with John Cheyne, described the pathologic type of breathing known as Cheyne-Stokes respiration.

The eventual triumphs of twentieth century medicine and surgery wouldn't have been possible without two other nineteenth century developments: anesthesia and antisepsis. In 1799, Sir Humphrey Davy wrote about the effect of nitrous oxide, noting that it was capable of "destroying pain and might probably be used with advantage in surgical operations." Nitrous oxide was used in dentistry in America in the 1840s. The recreational use of ether became popular at "ether frolics" in England after Michael Faraday noted that ether had a similar effect to nitrous oxide, or "laughing gas." Ether was first used for surgical anesthesia in 1842 by Crawford Long, a country practitioner in Georgia, who published an account of his discovery in 1849. In England, the first major operation using ether as an anesthetic took place at University College Hospital, London, in 1846. A painting formerly hanging in the Wellcome Historical Medical Museum depicts the administration of ether to a thirty-six-year-old butler named Frederick Churchill as the surgeon, Robert Liston, prepares to amputate his leg above the knee.

When the use of anesthetics was extended to women in childbirth, there was an outcry from some clergy and physicians in England who thundered that the Bible required women to suffer. The book of Genesis proclaimed: "in sorrow thou shalt bring forth children." Furthermore it was proposed, preposterously, that a woman's sufferings in labor were responsible for mother love. These misogynists alleged that anesthesia would "rob God of the deep earnest cries" of women in labor. Many physicians, however, swore by the use of painkillers during labor and delivery. Queen Victoria put an end to this battle after receiving chloroform from Dr. John Snow during her eighth confinement. She wrote that he "gave that blessed Chloroform & the effect was soothing, quieting & delightful beyond measure." She refused to accept that she should "bear cheerfully" pain that could be eliminated. Her regal acceptance paved the way for her subjects to avail themselves of obstetric anesthesia.

The horrible sufferings of surgical patients were alleviated by the introduction of anesthesia, but the other great scourge—infection—continued to claim many lives until the discoveries of Joseph Lister. As a student at University College Hospital, Lister had witnessed the operation on Frederick Churchill. Pasteur had already demonstrated that fermentation in wine was brought about by microscopic organisms and Lister deduced that wound infections were caused by similar agents. He experimented with various methods of destroying these organisms and eventually selected carbolic acid. He applied this treatment not only to wounds but also to dressings, surgical instruments, and the hands that dressed wounds. He published his results in *The Lancet* in 1867. Although his recommendations were met with hostility in some quarters, he eventually won over his critics and the era of surgical antisepsis was ushered in, saving countless lives.

Modern cardiology had its inception in the late nineteenth and early twentieth century. Augustus Waller (1859–1922), a general practitioner in London, recorded the electrical activity of the heart, laying the groundwork for the invention of the electrocardiogram. Sir Lauder Brunton (1844–1916) discovered the utility of nitrates in the treatment of angina pectoris, and to this day nitroglycerin is a mainstay of therapy. Pierre Potain (1825–1901), a French clinician, introduced the use of the sphygmomanometer to measure blood pressure. In 1912, James Herrick published one of the earliest accounts of a heart attack in the *Journal of the American Medical Association*. In his article, *Clinical Features of Sudden Obstruction of the Coronary Arteries* he described the symptoms of heart attack and noted that nearly all the cases he had seen were in men past the middle age.

Once again, wars proved a stimulus for the advancement of medicine. The twentieth century's widespread conflicts stimulated the growth of plastic surgery, the discovery of antibiotics, and the development of blood and plasma banks. Governments recognized the advantages that accrued from medical research and began to fund it on a hitherto unimaginable scale. Advances in cardiology and cardiac surgery were particularly breathtaking. Complete heart block, during which the heart rate drops to dangerously low levels, was effectively treated with an implanted pacemaker for the first time in 1959. This took place in Sweden when Ake Senning implanted a pacemaker developed by Rune Elmqvist.

Valvular disease of the heart was attacked surgically beginning in the 1920s. By the 1940s, physicians were turning their attention to congenital heart disease (cardiac malformations that are present in babies at birth). A young American pediatrician, Helen Taussig, in collaboration with Alfred Blalock, a cardiac surgeon, pioneered successful procedures to help babies with congenital heart defects. Their inability to stop the heart while operating without killing the patient kept the correction of the most serious defects tantalizingly out of reach.

In 1946, Dr. Arthur Vineberg reported on a new procedure to increase blood supply to the hearts of dogs with experimentally blocked coronary arteries. He took the internal mammary artery, implanted it into the heart muscle, and showed that new blood vessels formed in the area supplied by the blocked artery. The Vineberg operation was then performed on humans but was quickly superseded by a more effective operation made possible by two great advances: the heart-lung machine and coronary angiography.

As we noted in Chapter 11, during the 1950s surgeons and engineers working in several centers perfected the heart-lung machine. This device allowed surgeons to stop the heart while maintaining circulation by means of an external pump. Now they could replace or repair valves, cut out scars, and repair congenital defects. In 1962, Drs. Sones and Shirey of the Cleveland Clinic reported on a new way to diagnose coronary artery disease. Cine coronary arteriography, as they termed it, allowed physicians to take x-ray moving pictures of the arteries supplying the heart. The heart-lung machine and coronary angiography laid the groundwork for a great leap forward in the treatment of coronary artery disease: coronary artery bypass grafting (CABG).

In 1964, Dr. Michael DeBakey and his colleagues removed a length of vein from the leg and attached the proximal portion to the aorta and the distal portion to the diseased coronary artery beyond its obstruction, ushering in the modern era of cardiovascular surgery. The names of Michael DeBakey and Christian Barnard (who performed the first heart transplant in 1967) became almost as familiar to the general public as those of Joe DiMaggio and Marilyn Monroe.

The next great leap forward in cardiovascular therapeutics occurred in Switzerland in 1977, when Dr. Andreas Gruentzig performed the first balloon angioplasty to open up a blocked coronary artery in a 38-year-old man who suffered from angina pectoris. The golden age of cardiology had arrived.

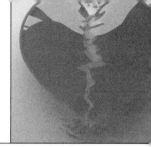

Chapter 15

Resources On- and Off-Line

There are many Web sites that you can consult to obtain information about cardiac disease. Several are aimed specifically at women. These URLs may prove helpful to you:

The Web site of the American Heart Association, *www.americanheart.org* and their program for women, Go Red For Women, *www.goredforwomen.org*.

The American Heart Association (AHA) has chapters in every state. The AHA funds cardiovascular disease research and is actively engaged in community education. For example, they sponsor courses in cardiopulmonary resuscitation (CPR). They publish educational pamphlets and cookbooks. The AHA is involved in lobbying Congress to join the fight against heart attacks and strokes. Their Go Red For Women program has a near-term goal of a 25% reduction in coronary heart disease and stroke risk by 2010. The AHA is a sponsor of the National Wear Red Day, in February, to increase awareness of heart disease in women.

The National Institutes of Health's National Heart, Lung and Blood Institute (NHLBI) has a Web site at *www.nhlbi.nih.gov*. In 2002 the NHLBI kicked off the Heart Truth Program with its symbol, the Red Dress. Its aim was to increase awareness of heart disease among women and it has been a huge success. Awareness that heart disease is the number one killer of women increased from 34% in 2000 to 57% in 2006. The Web site can be found at *www.nhlbi.nih.gov/health/hearttruth*.

The Women's Heart Foundation is a non-profit, non-governmental organization that designs and implements demonstration projects for the prevention of heart disease. It was founded by Bonnie Arkus, RN, who lost her own mother to heart disease. The Women's Heart Foundation is a charitable organization dedicated to improving the survival and quality of life for women with heart disease through the promotion of health literacy in gender care. (I am serving as Chief Medical Advisor of the Women's Heart Foundation 2006–2008.) The Web site can be found at *www.womensheart.org*.

Speaking of Women's Health is a non-profit foundation whose mission is "Saving Lives Through Education." Founded by Dianne Dunkelman in 1995, the foundation has grown exponentially. It sponsors regional conferences, newsletters, television programs, books, two minority health programs, and a very informative Web site. I am a member of Speaking of Women's Health National Advisory Panel. The Web site can be found at *www.speakingofwomenshealth.com*.

Offline, the American Heart Association publishes educational pamphlets and cookbooks. There are chapters in every state and you can contact your local chapter to obtain educational material and information about community education courses and events.

If there is a medical school in your area, chances are that one or more of the teaching hospitals affiliated with the school sponsors community education programs. Even if your local hospital isn't affiliated with a medical school, it may have such programs. Call your hospital and ask to speak to the community affairs office.

When it comes to heart disease, ignorance is not bliss, it can be downright deadly. Become a heart-wise woman and you'll improve your chances of living a long and healthy life.

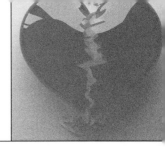

Afterword

The 2000 census results counted more than 143 million women living in the United States. More of these women will die of cardiovascular disease than of any other cause. In the year 2000, 13% of the female population of the United States was 65 or older, the age when cardiovascular disease becomes increasingly common. Since 1984, more women than men have died of heart disease each year in the United States. And yet the lay public, and even physicians, persist in believing that cardiac disease primarily affects men. In a 1995 Gallup poll, four out of five women and nearly one-third of primary care physicians didn't know that heart disease is the leading cause of death in women. With increased emphasis on educating women and the medical profession, these numbers have improved dramatically. But pockets of ignorance persist.

It's my fervent hope that the information in this book will help prevent the tragic situation I described in the introduction. Atherosclerosis can be ravaging your blood vessels at this very moment, even if you have no symptoms. Know your risk factors, and take the necessary steps to control them. Don't wait for some miracle drug to come along that will clean out your arteries after you've neglected them for years. It's not going to happen.

I hope this book will motivate you to take those all-important steps towards better health: don't smoke; exercise for 30 to 50 minutes most days; eat a balanced, heart-healthy diet; maintain a normal body weight; get regular check-ups; and take the medicines your physician prescribes if you have high blood pressure, diabetes, or high blood lipids. These steps are simple and doable, but no one can do them for you. As a woman, you probably take better care of your loved ones than you do of yourself. It's time to devote that same level of care to your own health. Get going and good luck.

Glossary

Abdominal or central obesity: Abnormal collection of fat in the abdomen that increases the risk of atherosclerosis; also called **visceral obesity.**

Ablation: The process of destroying tissue; for example ablation may be used to destroy an area in the heart that is causing an abnormal heart rhythm.

Alcoholic cardiomyopathy: A condition in which the heart muscle is damaged by excessive intake of alcohol.

Aliskerin: A direct renin inhibitor used to treat high blood pressure. Also called **Tekturna.**

Amino acids: The building blocks of proteins.

Ambrisentan: A medicine used to treat primary pulmonary hypertension. Also called **Letairis.**

Amiodarone: A medicine used in the treatment of certain abnormal heart rhythms. Also called **Cordarone.**

Amlodipine: A medicine used to treat high blood pressure and angina. Also called **Norvasc.**

Anasarca: Generalized edema or fluid retention.

Aneurysm: A weakened, bulging area in the heart or a blood vessel.

Angina pectoris: A symptom that often occurs when the heart muscle is starved for oxygen; usually felt as a squeezing, burning, or pressing discomfort in the chest or elsewhere in the upper body; it is usually brought on by exertion or stress and goes away in a few minutes with rest or relaxation.

Angiogram: A study in which dye is injected into a blood vessel and pictures are taken; also called **angiography.**

Angioplasty: Any intervention used to increase the opening or lumen of an artery.

Angiotensin converting enzyme inhibitor: A class of medicines used to treat high blood pressure and congestive heart failure.

Angiotensin receptor blocker: A class of medicine used to treat high blood pressure and congestive heart failure.

Anticoagulant: A medicine that makes the blood less likely to clot.

Antioxidant: A substance that combats the process of oxidation (when oxygen combines with another element).

Aorta: The main artery that leaves the left side of the heart.

Aortic regurgitation: A leaking of the aortic valve; also called **aortic insufficiency.**

Aortic stenosis: A narrowing of the aortic valve.

Aortic valve: The one-way valve between the pumping chamber on the left side of the heart (left ventricle) and the aorta.

Arrhythmia: An abnormality of the heart rhythm.

Arteriography: An angiogram of an artery; also called an **arteriogram.**

Arteriosclerosis: Hardening of the arteries.

Artery: A blood vessel that carries oxygenated blood.

Atenolol: A medicine used to treat angina and high blood pressure. Also called **Tenormin.**

Atherosclerosis: A form of arteriosclerosis in which plaque deposits build up in arteries.

Atrial fibrillation: An arrhythmia in which the atria beat very fast and irregularly, causing the pulse to be rapid and irregular; it increases the risk of stroke.

Atrial septal defect (ASD): A hole in the wall (septum) between the right and left atrium; one of the more common congenital defects (defects with which you are born).

Atrium (*pl.* atria): The upper, receiving chambers of the heart.

Automatic implantable cardiac defibrillator (AICD): A device that is inserted in the chest (usually through a vein) into the right side of the heart; it detects certain abnormal heart rhythms and delivers a shock to the heart to stop the arrhythmia.

Bacterial endocarditis: A bacterial infection of one or more heart valves.

Balloon catheter: A thin, hollow tube with an inflatable balloon on the end that can be inserted into an artery to open blockages.

Beta-blockers: A class of medicines used to treat angina, high blood pressure, and, sometimes, abnormal heart rhythms.

Bicuspid aortic valve: A congenital deformity of the aortic valve in which the valve has two cusps instead of the normal three.

Bisoprolol: A beta-blocker used to treat angina, congestive heart failure, and high blood pressure. Also called **Zebeta.**

Body Mass Index (BMI): A measure derived by dividing weight in kilograms by height in meters squared; normal values are between 18.5 and 24.9.

Bosentan: a medicine used to treat primary pulmonary hypertension. Also called **Tracleer**.

Bradycardia: An abnormal heart rhythm in which the heart beats too slowly; also called bradyarrhythmia.

Bruit: An abnormal sound heard over an artery that may indicate a blockage.

Buproprion: A medicine used to help alleviate symptoms of smoking withdrawal. Also called **Zyban**.

Calcific aortic stenosis: A form of aortic stenosis in which calcium builds up in the aortic valve; tends to occur in the elderly.

Calcium channel blockers: A class of medicines used to treat angina, high blood pressure, and, sometimes, abnormal heart rhythms.

Candesartan: A medicine used to treat high blood pressure and congestive heart failure. Also called **Atacand**.

Capillaries: The smallest blood vessels; they can only be seen with a microscope; the blood vessels from which oxygen is given up by the blood to the tissues.

Carbohydrates: Molecules that are made up of carbon, hydrogen, and oxygen; one of the major food classes.

Cardiac catheterization: A diagnostic procedure in which catheters (thin hollow tubes) are inserted into the heart from the arteries and/or veins to collect information about the heart's function.

Cardiac MRI: A non-invasive way to obtain information about the heart and its function.

Cardiac resynchronization therapy (CRT): A method of treating certain forms of heart failure with a special pacemaker called a biventricular pacemaker.

Cardiomyopathy: A condition in which the heart muscle is weakened or abnormal; it can have many causes including alcohol abuse, certain familial diseases, high blood pressure, diabetes, obesity, and prior heart attacks.

Cardiopulmonary bypass (CPB): The taking over of the circulation and oxygenation of the blood by a heart-lung machine during open heart surgery.

Cardiovascular: Relating to the heart and blood vessels.

Cardioversion: A procedure in which an electric shock is delivered to the heart, usually through the chest wall, to end an abnormal heart rhythm.

Carvedilol: A beta blocker medicine used to treat high blood pressure and heart failure. Also called **Coreg**.

Catheter: A long, thin, flexible, hollow tube, which is used in the study of the heart and blood vessels.

Cholesterol: A waxy substance found in every cell of the body that is important in the manufacture of many hormones; high levels of cholesterol increase the risk of atherosclerosis.

Cholestyramine: A medicine used to treat high blood levels of cholesterol; belongs to the class of medicines called "bile acid sequestrants" because they bind to bile in the intestines; also called **Questran.**

Chylomicron: Blood fat formed from dietary fat; very high levels can cause attacks of inflammation in the pancreas.

Cigarette smoking: A socially acceptable form of suicide; a major cause of atherosclerosis, heart attack, and stroke.

Click: An abnormal heart sound; may be heard in a common disorder of the mitral valve called mitral valve prolapse or "floppy" mitral valve.

Clopidogrel: A blood thinner commonly prescribed for people after angioplasty or for people at risk for heart attack or stroke. Also called **Plavix.**

Clot: A clump of blood that has solidified as a result of a complex process involving platelets and various proteins.

Coarctation of the aorta: A congenital defect that causes a narrowing of the aorta in the upper chest and high blood pressure; may be associated with a bicuspid aortic valve.

Colestipol: A bile acid sequestrant used to treat high blood levels of cholesterol. Also called **Colestid.**

Computerized tomography (CT): A special kind of x-ray in which a computer generates pictures of "slices" of the body and its organs.

Conduction system: The electrical system of the heart; the electric impulses that travel through the conduction system prompt the heart to contract and pump blood.

Congenital: Something with which you are born.

Constrictive pericarditis: A condition in which the lining of the heart becomes thickened and rigid and interferes with the heart's ability to function.

Contraceptive: A medicine or device that prevents pregnancy.

Coronary angiogram: A study in which dye is injected into the arteries supplying the heart to determine if they have any blockages; usually performed in conjunction with a cardiac catheterization; also called **coronary arteriography** or **coronary angiography.**

Coronary artery: An artery that supplies the heart muscle; there are usually two, the right coronary artery and the left coronary artery; they are the first branches of the aorta after it leaves the left side of the heart.

Coronary artery bypass graft surgery (CABG): An operation in which the surgeon uses veins or arteries to bypass blockages in the arteries supplying the heart.

Coronary artery disease (CAD): Disease of the arteries supplying the heart muscle; usually involves blockages caused by the build-up of atherosclerotic plaque.

C-reactive protein: A blood marker for inflammation; when elevated, it is a risk factor for atherosclerosis.

CT angiography (CTA): A special form of x-ray examination that can detect plaque in coronary arteries.

Cyanosis: A blue discoloration of the skin due to insufficient oxygen in the blood.

Defibrillation: The application of an electric shock to the heart to stop an abnormal heart rhythm.

Diabetes: A disease in which insulin, which regulates blood sugar levels, is either lacking (type 1 or insulin-dependent diabetes) or, more commonly, is elevated but less effective (type 2 or non-insulin-dependent diabetes).

Diastole: That portion of the heart cycle where the heart is relaxed.

Diastolic blood pressure: The pressure in the arteries while the heart is relaxed; it is the lower of the two numbers your doctor measures when taking your blood pressure.

Digoxin: A form of the medicine digitalis that is used to increase the pumping strength of the heart or to slow the pulse in atrial fibrillation. Also called **Lanoxin.**

Diltiazem: A medicine used to treat angina, high blood pressure, coronary artery spasm, and certain abnormal heart rhythms. Also called **Cardizem, Cartia, Tiazac, Dilacor.**

Dipyridamole: A blood thinner; sometimes used in nuclear stress tests. Also called **Persantine.**

Diuretics: Medicines that increase urine output that are used in the treatment of high blood pressure and heart failure.

Dyslipidemia: Abnormal levels of blood fats; also called **dyslipoproteinemia.**

Dyspnea: Shortness of breath.

Echocardiogram: A test that uses sound waves to construct images of the heart and valves; also called **echocardiography** or **ultrasonography.**

Edema: Abnormal swelling of the tissues; usually seen in the legs in conditions such as heart failure.

Electrocardiogram (EKG): A graphic display of the electrical activity of the heart.

Electron beam tomography: A specialized x-ray study that's useful in measuring the amount of calcium in the coronary arteries.

Electrophysiologic study (EPS): A special procedure performed in a laboratory in which catheters are inserted into the heart to test the heart's electrical system; sometimes an ablation of an abnormal focus of electrical activity is done during EPS.

Embolus (*pl.* emboli): A clot that has broken off and traveled from one place in the body to another; also called an **embolism.**

Enalapril: A medicine used to treat high blood pressure and heart failure. Also called **Vasotec.**

Endocarditis: Infection or inflammation of the heart valves.

Epinephrine: A naturally occurring substance that is released in the body in response to stress; also called **adrenaline.**

Eplerenone: A diuretic that is used in the treatment of high blood pressure and congestive heart failure. Also called **Inspra.**

Epoprostenol: An intravenous medicine used to treat primary pulmonary hypertension. Also called **Flolan.**

Eprosartan: A medicine used to treat high blood pressure. Also called **Teveten.**

Estrogen: One of the female reproductive hormones.

Estrogen replacement therapy (ERT): The treatment of women after menopause with estrogen.

Exercise stress test: A test that uses exercise to evaluate whether a symptom such as chest pain is being caused by coronary narrowing; also called an **exercise tolerance test.**

Ezetimibe: A medicine used to treat high cholesterol. Also called **Zetia.**

Fatty acids: Substances found in food that are used by the body to generate energy.

Fatty streak: An early sign of atherosclerosis.

Femoral artery: A large artery in the groin that supplies blood to the leg; it is commonly punctured in the course of a cardiac catheterization so that catheters can be inserted and advanced into the heart.

Fenofibrate: A medicine used to treat high triglycerides and high cholesterol; also called **Tricor.**

Fibric acid derivatives: A class of medicines used to treat high blood lipids, particularly high triglycerides; also called **fibrates.**

Fibrinogen: A substance involved in blood clotting; high levels are associated with an increased risk of atherosclerosis.

Fibromuscular dysplasia: A specific form of narrowing that occurs in the artery supplying the kidney; more common in young women than men.

Flecainide: A medicine used to treat abnormal heart rhythms. Also called **Tambocor.**

Fluvastatin: A medicine used to treat high blood cholesterol. Also called **Lescol.**

Folic acid: A B vitamin that is used to treat high levels of homocysteine; also called **folate.**

Furosemide: A diuretic used to treat heart failure and high blood pressure. Also called **Lasix.**

Gemfibrozil: A medicine used to treat high blood levels of triglycerides. Also called **Lopid.**

Glucose: A simple sugar that is used in the body to generate energy.

Heart failure: A condition in which the heart is unable to pump enough blood for the body's needs; can have many causes; also called **congestive heart failure.**

Hemochromatosis: A familial disease in which abnormal amounts of iron are stored in the tissues of the body; can be the cause of heart and liver failure.

Hemoptysis: The coughing up of blood.

Hemorrhage: Abnormal bleeding.

Heparin: A blood thinner or anticoagulant; must be given by injection.

High-density lipoprotein (HDL): "Good" cholesterol; it helps protect against atherosclerosis.

Holter monitor: A device that records the EKG for 24 hours; used to determine the cause of fainting or palpitations.

Homocysteine: An amino acid that is a risk factor for atherosclerosis when its level is elevated.

Hormone replacement therapy (HRT): The treatment, with estrogen and progesterone, of women who are past menopause.

Hydralazine: A medicine used to treat high blood pressure. Also called **Apresoline.**

Hydrochlorothiazide: A diuretic used to treat high blood pressure. Also called **Hydrodiuril, Esidrix.**

Hypercholesterolemia: High blood levels of cholesterol.

Hyperglycemia: High blood sugar.

Hyperlipidemia: High levels of cholesterol and/or triglyceride; also called **hyperlipoproteinemia.**

Hypertension: High blood pressure.

Hypertrophic cardiomyopathy: A condition in which the walls of the heart are abnormally thickened.

Hypothyroidism: A disease in which the thyroid is underactive.

Iloprost: A medicine taken as a nasal spray to treat primary pulmonary hypertension. Also called **Ventavis.**

Infective endocarditis (IE): Infection, usually bacterial, of one or more cardiac valves.

Inferior vena cava: A large vein that brings blood from the lower body to the right side of the heart.

Insulin: A hormone made by the pancreas that regulates the level of glucose in the blood.

Interleukin: A marker of inflammation.

Intermediate-density lipoprotein (IDL): A blood fat that is formed by the breakdown of very low density lipoprotein.

Intravascular ultrasound (IVUS): A way to determine the amount of plaque in a blood vessel by using sound waves. Usually performed during the course of coronary angiography.

Intima: The innermost layer of an artery; it is the first line of defense protecting the artery from harmful substances in the blood.

Irbesartan: A medicine used to treat high blood pressure and diabetic kidney disease. Also called **Avapro.**

Ischemia: A condition in which the blood supply to an organ is not sufficient for the organ's needs.

Isosorbide: A medicine that dilates blood vessels; used in the treatment of angina. Also called **Isordil.**

Isotope: Radioactive chemicals that undergo spontaneous disintegration resulting in the emission of certain types of rays, including x-rays.

Left Anterior Descending Artery: One of the two major branches of the left coronary artery.

Left Circumflex Artery: One of the two major branches of the left coronary artery.

Left Internal Mammary Artery (LIMA): An artery in the chest that is often used by cardiac surgeons to bypass blockages in the coronary arteries.

Left ventricle: The pumping chamber on the left side of the heart.

Left ventricular hypertrophy: Abnormal thickening of the muscle in the left ventricle.

Lipid: Another word for blood fats.

Lipoprotein: A blood fat joined to a protein.

Lisinopril: A medicine used to treat high blood pressure and heart failure. Also called **Zestril** or **Prinivil.**

Long QT Syndrome: An inherited disorder which increases the risk of abnormal (and sometimes fatal) heart rhythms.

Losartan: A medicine used to treat high blood pressure and heart failure. Also called **Cozaar.**

Lovastatin: The first "statin" medicine to be approved in the United States; used to treat high cholesterol. Also called **Mevacor.**

Low-density lipoprotein (LDL): The "bad" cholesterol; high levels increase the risk of atherosclerosis.

Lp(a): An altered blood fat which when elevated may be a risk factor for atherosclerosis.

Lumen: The passage in an artery or vein through which blood flows.

Magnetic resonance imaging (MRI): A way to visualize organs in the body using magnetic energy.

Mediterranean diet: A diet rich in olive oil, colorful fruits and vegetables, whole grains, legumes (beans), and seafood but low in meat; consumed in the countries bordering the Mediterranean Sea; considered the healthiest diet in the world.

Medroxyprogesterone acetate: A form of progesterone, one of the female reproductive hormones. Also called **Provera.**

Menopause: The cessation of menses for one year; occurs at an average age of 52.

Menses: The monthly loss of blood from the uterus of a woman during her reproductive years.

Metabolic syndrome: A clustering of abnormalities, including abdominal obesity, high blood pressure, insulin resistance, abnormal clotting, and abnormal blood fats that greatly increase the risk of atherosclerosis.

Metoprolol: A beta-blocker used to treat angina, high blood pressure, heart failure, and certain abnormal heart rhythms; also called **Toprol** or **Lopressor.**

Minoxidil: A medicine used to treat high blood pressure which is unresponsive to other agents. Also called **Loniten.**

Mitral regurgitation: A condition in which blood leaks back from the left ventricle to the left atrium when the heart contracts; also called **mitral insufficiency.**

Mitral stenosis: A condition in which the mitral valve opening becomes narrowed, obstructing blood flow from the left atrium to the left ventricle.

Mitral valve: A one-way valve on the left side of the heart that is found between the left atrium and the left ventricle.

Mitral valve prolapse (MVP): A condition in which the mitral valve attachments are lax and the leaflets themselves are billowy, allowing the mitral valve leaflets to bulge into the left atrium when the left ventricle contracts; also called a **floppy mitral valve.**

Multivessel CAD: Coronary blockages involving more than one coronary artery.

Murmurs: Abnormal sounds that are usually caused by turbulent blood flow, as when a heart valve is narrowed or leaky.

Myocardial infarction: Death of heart muscle due to interruption of its blood supply; usually caused by the rupture of a plaque with clot formation that totally blocks blood supply to a portion of the heart; also called a heart attack.

Myocardial ischemia: A condition in which the heart muscle is not getting enough blood supply for its needs; usually caused by blockages in the arteries supplying the heart.

Myocarditis: Inflammation of the heart muscle.

Myocardium: A medical term for the heart muscle.

Myxoma: A cardiac tumor that usually arises in the left atrium.

Nadolol: A beta-blocker medicine used to treat angina, high blood pressure, and certain abnormal heart rhythms. Also called **Corgard.**

Nebivolol: A beta-blocker used to treat high blood pressure. Also called **Bystolic.**

Niacin: A B vitamin used to treat high triglycerides; also raises HDL cholesterol and lowers total and LDL cholesterol; also called **nicotinic acid** or **Niaspan.**

Nifedipine: A calcium channel blocker used to treat high blood pressure and angina. Also called **Procardia** or **Adalat.**

Nitrates: A class of medicines that dilate blood vessels; used to treat angina.

Nitroglycerin: The most commonly prescribed nitrate used to treat angina.

Nuclear stress test: A test using radioactive chemicals to detect areas of the heart which are not receiving adequate blood supply.

Obesity: A body mass index of 30.0 or above.

Olmesartan: a medicine used to treat high blood pressure. Also called **Benicar.**

Omega-3 fatty acids: Compounds found in fish, canola oil, and walnuts that protect against sudden cardiac death.

Omega-6 fatty acids: Compounds found in corn, safflower, and soybean oils that are required to form certain hormones.

Oral contraceptive: Pills that prevent pregnancy; usually a combination of an estrogen and a progesterone.

Orthopnea: Shortness of breath that occurs when lying down; usually a symptom of heart failure.

Orthostatic hypotension: A drop in blood pressure that occurs when moving from a lying or sitting position to a standing position.

Osteoporosis: A condition in which bones become thin and brittle; affects women more than men, especially after menopause.

Oxygen: An element that is necessary for life; carried in the blood and given up by blood in the capillaries to nourish all the tissues of the body.

P wave: A part of the electrocardiogram that is caused by electricity traveling through the atria.

Pacemaker: Natural pacemakers occur in the heart; if these fail, a doctor can insert an artificial pacemaker, which will stimulate the heart to beat.

Palpitations: A sensation of fluttering in the chest that is usually caused by extra heart beats or abnormal heart rhythms.

Parasympathetic nervous system: A part of the nervous system that usually causes the heart rate to slow and the blood pressure to drop.

Paroxysmal nocturnal dyspnea (PND): Attacks of waking up at night very short of breath; commonly a symptom of heart failure.

Percutaneous coronary intervention (PCI): Procedures in which various types of catheters and devices are used to improve blood flow to the heart.

Percutaneous transluminal coronary angioplasty (PTCA): A procedure in which a balloon-tipped catheter is inserted into a coronary artery in a narrowed area to dilate it and improve blood flow.

Pericardial effusion: An abnormal collection of fluid in the pericardial sac around the heart.

Pericardial tamponade: An abnormal collection of large amounts of fluid around the heart; can cause shock and death if severe.

Pericarditis: An inflammation or infection of the pericardium.

Pericardium: A sac that surrounds the heart; composed of two layers of cells.

Peripartum cardiomyopathy: A disease that occurs late in pregnancy or just after childbirth in which the heart muscle becomes weakened, thus causing heart failure.

Peripheral vascular disease: Atherosclerosis involving the arteries to the leg; when severe, it can lead to gangrene and amputation; also called **peripheral arterial disease**.

Phlebothrombosis: A clot that sits in a vein but does not cause inflammation.

Plant stanol esters: Compounds that block the absorption of cholesterol from the bowel.

Plaque: A build-up of material composed of lipids, smooth muscle cells, and white blood cells in the walls of arteries, eventually causing the artery to be narrowed.

Plasminogen: A naturally occurring molecule that is involved in dissolving clots.

Platelets: Microscopic elements in the blood that are involved in the formation of clots.

Pleura: The lining of the lungs; analogous to the pericardium.

Porcine valve: An artificial heart valve manufactured from pig tissue.

Positron emission tomography (PET scan): A radiologic test using isotopes that allows the metabolic activity of tissues to be measured.

Potassium: An element found in the blood and in cells; its levels are tightly regulated because levels that are either too high or too low can be dangerous.

Pravastatin: A statin medication used to treat high cholesterol. Also called **Pravachol**.

Prazosin: A medicine used to treat high blood pressure. Also called **Minipress**.

Premature contraction: A heartbeat coming sooner than normal; these can arise from the atria or the ventricle; also called a **premature beat**.

Primary Pulmonary Hypertension (PPH): A disease of unknown cause that affects women more than men and can lead to irreversible heart failure.

Prinzmetal angina (also called variant or vasospastic angina): Angina caused by a coronary artery going into spasm.

Procainamide: A medicine used to treat certain abnormal heart rhythms. Also called **Pronestyl** or **Procan.**

Progesterone: One of the female reproductive hormones.

Propranolol: A beta-blocker medicine used to treat angina and high blood pressure; also called **Inderal.**

Prosthetic heart valve: An artificial heart valve; can be made from animal tissue, plastic, or metal.

Protein: Compounds that contain amino acids; found in vegetables and meat.

Pulmonary: Relating to the lungs.

Pulmonary artery: The artery that conducts venous blood from the right ventricle to the lungs.

Pulmonic valve: A one-way valve between the right ventricle and the pulmonary artery.

Pulse: The impulse that the contraction of the heart causes; it can be felt over various arteries, including those in the neck, wrist, groin, and feet.

QRS complex: A deflection on the electrocardiogram caused by electricity traveling through the ventricles; also called a Q wave.

Quinidine: A medicine used to treat certain abnormal heart rhythms. Also called **Quinidex** or **Quinaglute.**

Radio-frequency ablation: The process of destroying abnormal tissue by applying radio waves that generate heat; usually done for abnormal heart rhythms.

Raloxifene: An estrogen-like medicine used to treat osteoporosis. Also called **Evista.**

Ranolazine: A medicine used to treat angina. Also called **Ranexa.**

Renal: Relating to the kidneys.

Renal artery stenosis: A narrowing in the artery supplying the kidney; can be a cause of high blood pressure.

Renovascular hypertension: High blood pressure caused by a narrowing of one or more of the arteries supplying the kidneys.

Restenosis: Recurrent narrowing of an artery after it has been dilated.

Rheumatic fever: A disease that causes thickening and malfunction of the heart valves; results from certain strep infections.

Right ventricle: The pumping chamber on the right side of the heart.

Risk factor: Any characteristic that increases an individual's chance of developing a disease.

Rosuvastatin: A medicine used to treat high cholesterol. Also called **Crestor.**

Salicylates: Aspirin-like medicines.

Septum: The wall between the right and left ventricles; also called the **intraventricular septum.**

Sildenafil: A medicine used to treat primary pulmonary hypertension. Also called **Revatio.** (When used to treat erectile dysfunction is called **Viagra.**)

Simvastatin: One of the statin medicines used to treat high cholesterol. Also called **Zocor.**

Sinus node: The normal pacemaker of the heart.

Sodium: An element found in blood and cells that is regulated by the kidneys within narrow limits; levels that are too high or too low can be dangerous.

Sotalol: A medicine used to treat certain abnormal heart rhythms. Also called **Betapace.**

Spiral CT: A special form of x-ray examination that can be used to help diagnose conditions like aortic dissection, and pulmonary embolus.

Spironolactone: A diuretic that is used in the treatment of high blood pressure and congestive heart failure; also called **Aldactone.**

ST segment: A portion of the electrocardiogram that is measured in exercise stress testing.

Statins: A class of medicines that is very effective in treating high cholesterol and decreasing the risk of heart attack, stroke, and cardiac death.

Stenosis: Narrowing or blockage of valves or blood vessels.

Stent: Wire mesh that is put into an artery after a stenosis has been dilated to help prevent acute reblockage.

Stroke: Death of brain cells due to an interruption of blood supply; also called cerebrovascular accident (CVA).

Sudden cardiac death: Death that occurs within minutes when the heart ceases to beat or beats too rapidly to maintain circulation.

Superior vena cava: The large vein that drains venous blood from the upper body into the right atrium.

Sympathetic nervous system: The part of the nervous system involved in the "fight or flight" reflex; generally causes the pulse and blood pressure to rise.

Syncope: Fainting.

Systole: The part of the heart's cycle in which the ventricles are contracting.

Tachycardia: An abnormally fast heart rate; also called a **tachyarrhythmia.**

Takotsubo cardiomyopathy: A form of cardiomyopathy which is often self-limited and affects women much more often than men.

Technetium: An isotope used in nuclear stress tests.

Telmisartan: A medicine used to treat high blood pressure. Also called **Micardis.**

Testosterone: A male reproductive hormone; also found in women but at lower levels than in men.

Thallium: An isotope used in nuclear stress tests.

Thrombolysis: The process by which clots are dissolved.

Thrombolytics: Medicines that dissolve clots.

Thrombophlebitis: A condition in which a clot forms in a vein and inflames it.

Thrombosis: The process of abnormal clot formation.

Thrombus (*pl.* thrombi): A clot occurring where it shouldn't be.

Ticlopidine: A blood thinner. Also called **Ticlid.**

Transesophogeal echocardiography (TEE): A procedure in which a scope is inserted into the esophagus (the tube leading from the mouth to the stomach) and ultrasound pictures of the heart are obtained.

Transmyocardial laser revascularization: A procedure to increase blood supply to the heart for people with severe angina who cannot have bypass surgery or angioplasty.

Triamterene: A diuretic. Also called **Dyrenium.**

Tricuspid regurgitation: Leakage of blood through the tricuspid valve back into the right atrium when the right ventricle contracts; also called **tricuspid insufficiency.**

Tricuspid stenosis: A narrowing of the tricuspid valve.

Tricuspid valve: The valve on the right side of the heart between the right atrium and the right ventricle.

Triglyceride: A blood fat; high levels increase the risk of atherosclerosis, particularly in women.

Valsartan: A medicine used to treat high blood pressure and heart failure. Also called **Diovan.**

Valves: Structures in the heart that keep the blood flowing in the correct direction.

Varenicline: A medicine used to help smokers quit. Also called **Chantix.**

Vasovagal syncope: The fancy medical term for the common fainting spell.

Veins: Blood vessels that carry blood that has given up oxygen to the tissues and taken up carbon dioxide from the tissues.

Ventricles: The pumping chambers in the heart; the right ventricle pumps blood to the lungs; the left ventricle pumps blood to the body.

Ventricular fibrillation: A rapidly fatal arrhythmia in which the heart quivers rather than contracts.

Ventricular tachycardia: An abnormally fast heart rhythm arising in the ventricle.

Verapamil: A calcium channel blocker used to treat angina, high blood pressure, and certain abnormal heart rhythms; also called **Isoptin, Calan,** or **Covera.**

Very low-density lipoprotein (VLDL): A lipoprotein that is the main carrier of triglycerides in the blood.

Warfarin: A blood thinner. Also called **Coumadin.**

Xanthoma: A collection of cholesterol in the skin or in a tendon.

Index

Italicized page locators indicate a figure; tables are noted with a *t*.

A

F

Fainting, 110–112
False negative tests, 118, 120
False positive tests, 118
Familial hypercholesterolemia, 23, 205
Faraday, Michael, 221
Fasting blood glucose level, 29–30
Fats, 57
"Fat Transport in Lipoproteins"
    (Levy and Fredrickson), 20
Fatty acids, 22
Fatty streaks, 11
FDA. *See* Food and Drug
    Administration
Felodipine, 146
Female heart transplant recipients, 182
Females. *See also* Gender bias;
    Women
        atrial septal defect and, 98
        coarctation of the aorta and, 99
Feminism, impact of, in medicine,
    190
Fenfluramine, 93, 101
Fenofibrate, 45, 159, 160
"Fen-phen," 93
Fiber, 56
Fibric acid derivatives, 43, 158–160
Fibrinogen, 16, 43
Fibromuscular dysplasia, 28
FIELD trial, 160
Fight or flight response, 111, 143
Fish consumption, fatty, 54
Fish oils, 54, 58, 162–163
Flecainide, 164
Flolan, 148
Fluvastatin, 157
Flynn, Mary, 53
Foam cells, 11
Folic acid (folate), 42
Food and Drug Administration, 59,
    60, 143, 157, 187
Fosamax, 77
Fosinopril, 142
Fourth National Health and
    Nutrition Examination Survey, 33

Framingham, Massachusetts, 13
Framingham risk score, components
    of, 16
Framingham Study, 21, 31, 34, 66, 107
    angina pectoris in women and,
        103, 104
    description of, 13–16
    fibrinogen and, 43
    Lp(a) and, 44, 45
Fredrickson, Donald, 20
Free fatty acids, 22
Fruits and vegetables, 54–55
Furosemide, 141

G

Gadolinium, 135–136
Galen, 211–212, 213, 216
Galiani, Alexandra, 215
Gall bladder disease, in overweight
    individuals, 35
Gemfibrozil, 159, 160
Gender
    angina pectoris and, 103, 104,
        105, 144
    aortic dissection and, 100
    atrial septal defect and, 98
    CABG and, 187
    coarctation of the aorta and, 99
    coronary artery bypass grafts
        and, 178–179
    diabetes, congestive heart
        failure and, 31
    exercise benefits and, 38–39
    exercise stress testing and, 127
    false positive ST depression
        and, 124
    heart and, 7
    homocysteine levels and, 42
    hypertension and, 26, 27
    mitral regurgitation and, 95
    myocardial infarction and, 107
    nicotine addiction and, 18
    obesity and, 33–34
    Primary Pulmonary
        Hypertension and, 100

Infection, of cardiac valves, 90
Infective endocarditis, 90
Inferior vena cavae, 1, 2
Inflammation
    Celsus and cardinal signs of,
        210–211
    plague formation and, 10–11
    smoking and markers for, 19
Inflammatory reaction, 45
Insoluble fiber, 56
Inspra, 141
Insulin-dependent diabetes, 30
Insulin sensitivity, exercise and, 38
Integrilin, 152
Interleukin, 45
Intermediate-density lipoprotein, 22
Intermittent claudication, 80
International Journal of
    Epidemiology, 19
Intima, 10
Intravascular ultrasound, 104, 131
Irbesartan, 143
Ischemia, 80, 102
Ischemic heart disease, 86
Islam, medical knowledge and, 212–214
Isoptin, 146
Isordil, 145
Isosorbide, 145
IVUS. *See* Intravascular ultrasound

J

Jews, public health and, 208
Johnson, Samuel, 219
Joint National Committee (JNC)
    on Detection, Evaluation, and
    Treatment of High Blood Pressure,
    82
Journal of the American College of
    Cardiology, 15, 193
Journal of the American Medical
    Association, 39, 40, 70, 71, 74, 77,
    125, 170, 223
Journeys in Divers Places (Paré), 217
Julius Caesar, 210
Juvenile diabetes, 30

K

Keys, Ancel, 54
Kidney disease, digoxin and, 140
Kidney disease, gadolinium and, 136
Koch, Robert, 221

L

Labetolol, 143
Labile hypertension, 26–27
Labor and delivery, anesthesia and,
    222
Lactose intolerance, 56
Laennec, Rene, 220
Lancet, The, 12, 153, 175, 223
Lanoxin, 140
Lasix, 141
"Laughing gas," 221
Lauterburg, Paul, 134
LDL receptor, 23
LDLs. *See* Low-density lipoproteins
Leaky valves
    fen-phen and, 93
    mitral, 95–96
    repairing, 176
Left anterior descending artery, 3
Left atria (atrium), 1, 2, 3
Left circumflex artery, 3
Left coronary artery, 3
Left internal mammary artery, 179
Left pulmonary artery, 3
Left ventricle, 1, 2, 3
Left ventricular angiogram, 132
Left ventricular hypertrophy, 27, 83
Lescol, 157
Letairis, 148
Levy, Robert I., 20, 21, 24
Lidocaine, 164
LIMA. *See* Left internal mammary
    artery
Lipid levels, genetic disorders and, 24
Lipid profiles, exercise and, 38
Lipid Research Clinic Program, 21
Lipids, 21, 57
Lipid transport system, 22
Lipitor, 157

Nebivolol, 143
Negative tests, 118
Nephrogenic fibrosing dermopathy, 136
Nephrogenic Systemic Fibrosis, 136
New England Journal of Medicine,
20, 32, 78, 193
NFD. *See* Nephrogenic fibrosing
dermopathy
NHANES III. *See* Third National
Health and Nutrition Examination
Survey
NHANES IV. *See* Fourth National
Health and Nutrition Examination
Survey
NHLBI. *See* National Heart, Lung,
and Blood Institute
Niacin, 45, 158, 161–162
high-density lipoproteins and, 25
side effects with, 161–162
Niaspan, 162
Nicorandil, 202
Nicotine, 18
Nicotine addiction, women and, 18
Nicotine patches, 20
Nifedipine, 146, 148
Nitrates, 144–145
Nitroglycerin, 144, 223
Nitrous oxide, 221
Nolvadex, 77
Non-insulin-dependent diabetes, 30
Normal weight, defined, 33
Normodyne, 143
Norpace, 164
North American Menopause Society,
76
Norvasc, 146, 148
NSF. *See* Nephrogenic Systemic
Fibrosis
Nuclear scans, interpreting, 126
Nuclear stress tests, 124–125, 127
gender bias and use of, 191
Nurses Health Study, 17, 19, 34, 40
Nurses Health Study II, 31

O

Obesity, 32–38
cardiovascular disease and, 34–35
epidemic of, 61
gender and, 33–34
hypertension and, 28–29, 84
prevalence of, 32–33
race, socioeconomic, and ethnic
differences related to, 35
as risk factor for cardiovascular
disease, 14
type 2 diabetes and, 30
Observational studies, 69
Obstetric anesthesia, history behind,
222
Off-pump bypass surgery, 180
Old Testament, 208
Olestra, 60
Olive oil, 54, 57
Olmesartan, 143
Omega-3 fatty acids, 58
Omega-6 fatty acids, 58
Oral contraceptives
blood pressure checks and use
of, 27
high blood pressure and, 84
smoking and, 18
Organic nitrates, 144
Ornish, Dean, 52
Orthopnea, 94
Orthostatic hypotension, 111
Osteoarthritis, in overweight
individuals, 35
Osteoporosis
exercise and, 40
treatment of, 77
Ovaries, 15, 66
Overweight. *See also* Obesity
defined, 33
hypertension and, 27
Oxidation, 60
Oxygen, 1

P

Pacemakers, 102, 205
  biventricular, 187
  early, 223
  electromagnetic energy and,
    186
  parts of, 183–184
Palpitations, 28, 91, 110
Paradoxical embolism, 98
Paré, Ambrose, 216, 217
Paroxysmal nocturnal dyspnea, 81,
  94, 109
Partially hydrogenated vegetable oil,
  59
Pasteur, Louis, 221, 222
Patent foramen ovale, 98–99, 171
PCI. *See* Percutaneous coronary
  intervention
PCO. *See* Polycystic ovary syndrome
Percutaneous coronary angioplasty,
  gender bias and use of, 192
Percutaneous coronary intervention,
  167
    benefits with, 173
    women and, 170–171
Percutaneous transluminal coronary
  angioplasty, 167
Pericardial knock, 85
Pericardial rub, 85
Pericardial sac, 84
Pericardial tamponade, 85
Pericarditis, 84, 85, 108
Pericardium, 3, 84
Perindopril, 142
Peripartum cardiomyopathy, 87
Peripheral vascular disease, 19
Persantine, 125, 150
PET scan. *See* Positron emission
  tomography scan
PFO. *See* Patent foramen ovale
Phlebothrombosis, 43
Physical activity, 38–41

Physical inactivity
  central obesity and, 34
  as risk factor for cardiovascular
    disease, 14
Physician bias, referral patterns for
  men and women and, 193
Physicians
  Muslim, 213
  trust issues and, 198–199, 200
  women, in Rome, 210
Placebo control group, 68, 69
Plant stanol esters, 59–60
Plaque, 10, 13
  buildup of, in coronary arteries,
    11
Plasma banks, 223
Plasminogen, 44
Plastic surgery, 223
Platelets, 43
  aspirin and, 148
Plavix, 150, 169
Plendil, 146
Pleuritic pain, 108
Pliny the Elder, 210
Pluripotent stem cells, 202
PND. *See* Paroxysmal nocturnal
  dyspnea
Pneumonia, 108
Polycystic ovary syndrome, 31
Polysaccharides, 56
Polyunsaturated fats, 57, 58
Pompeii, 210
Pondimin, 93
Positive tests, 118, 120
Positron emission tomography scan,
  125
Postmenopausal Estrogen/Progestin
  Interventions (PEPI) Trial, 70, 72
Potain, Pierre, 223
Potassium channel activators, angina
  treatment and, 201–202
Potassium-rich foods, diuretics and,
  141

PPH. *See* Primary Pulmonary
  Hypertension
Pravachol, 154, 157
Pravastatin, 154, 157
Prazosin, 146
Predictive value, 119, 120
Prednisone, cardiac transplantations
  and, 182
Pregnancy
  fibric acid derivatives and, 160
  statins and, 158
Premarin, 66, 73, 74
Premature contractions, 91, 129
Premenopausal women, lower
  incidence of heart disease in, 66,
  68
Prempro, 74, 75
Prevalence, 14, 120
Primary prevention trials, 69
Primary Pulmonary Hypertension,
  100–101, 148
Prinivil, 142
Procainamide, 164
Procardia, 146, 148
Progesterone, 68, 70, 72, 75
Progestins, 66, 68, 72
Pronestyl, 164
Propranolol, 143, 144
Proteins, 42, 56–57
PROVE-IT TIMI 22 study, 154
PSEs. *See* Plant stanol esters
PTCA. *See* Percutaneous
  transluminal coronary angioplasty
Puel, J., 168
Pulmonary alveoli, 2
Pulmonary artery, 2, 3
Pulmonary capillaries, 2, 112
Pulmonary embolus (emboli), 43,
  96, 98
    CT imaging and, 133
    pleuritic chest pain and, 108
Pulmonary veins, 2
Pulmonic valves, 2, 89
P wave, 121, *122*

Q

QRS complex, 121, *122*
Questran, 160
Quinapril, 142
Quinidine (Quinidex), 164

R

Race. *See also* African-Americans;
  Ethnicity; Whites
    cardiovascular health and, 82
    diabetes and, 30
    exercise and, 38
    hypertension and, 26, 83
    obesity and, 35
Racial bias, heart treatment and,
  194–195
Radioactive isotopes, 124
Radiofrequency ablation, 172
    gender bias and, 192–193
Raloxifene (Evista), 77, 78
Raloxifene Use for The Heart, 78
Ramipril, 142
Randomized, double-blind, placebo-
  controlled study, 69
Ranolazine (Ranexa), 145
Rebecca (woman physician at
  Salerno), 214
Redux, 93
Referral services, hospital, 199
Regurgitant valves, 89
Renaissance, medicine during, 216–217
Renal artery stenosis, types of, 27–28
Renin, 147
Renovascular hypertension, 28
ReoPro, 152
Restenosis, 167–168
    lessening risk of, 205
Resting heart rates, in men *vs.* women, 7
Revatio, 148
Rhazes, 213
Rheumatic fever, 89–90, 92, 95

Therapeutic alliance, with physician, 200
Therapeutic Lifestyle Changes (TLC) Diet, nutrient composition of, 53
Thiazide diuretics, 158
Third National Health and Nutrition Examination Survey, 32
Thrombolysis, 43
Thrombolytics, 43, 151–152, 171
Thrombophlebitis, 43
Thrombosis, 42–43
Thrombus, 42
Thyroid replacement, 86
TIA. See Transient ischemic attack
Tiazac, 146
Ticlopidine (Ticlid), 150
Tikosyn, 164
TMR. See Transmyocardial revascularization with laser
TNF. See Tumor necrosis factor
Tobacco industry, 16
Toprol, 143
"Torsade de points," 164
Totipotent stem cells, 202
Tracleer, 148
Trandate, 143
Trandolapril, 142
Transesophageal echocardiogram, 127–128
Trans-fatty acids, 53, 58–59
Transient ischemic attack, 80
Transmyocardial revascularization with laser, 181
Transplanted hearts, complications related to, 182–183
Transplanted organs, immune response and, 87
Transthoracic echocardiogram, 127
Treatment to New Targets trial, 155
Triamterene, 141
Tricor, 159, 160
Tricuspid regurgitation, 96
Tricuspid valves, 1, 2, 89
Triglycerides
    beta-blockers and, 143
    carbohydrate-rich diets and, 25
    Mediterranean diet and, 55

smoking and elevation of, 18
statins and, 157
Trotula (woman physician at Salerno), 214
True negative tests, 118
True positive tests, 118
Trust, in physicians, 198–199, 200
Tuberculosis, 213
Tumor necrosis factor, 45
Twain, Mark, 117
T wave, 121, *122*
IIb/IIIa inhibitors, 152
Type 1 diabetes, 30
    coronary artery disease and, 31
Type 2 diabetes, 30
    obesity and, 34
    polycystic ovary syndrome and, 31
Type III hyperlipidemia, 159

U

United Network for Organ Sharing, 182
United States, female population in, 231
United States Public Health Service, 20
Univasc, 142
Uterine cancer, 68, 73

V

Vagus nerve, 111–112
Valsartan, 143
Valvular heart disease, 175
Valvulotomy, 95
Varenicline (Chantix), 20
Vasotec, 142
Vasovagal syncope, 111, 112
Vegetables and fruits, 54–55
Veins, 1
Ventavis, 148
Ventricles, 1, *2*, *3*
Ventricular fibrillation, 18, 102, 185
Ventricular septal defect, 99
Verapamil, 146, 163
Very low-density lipoproteins, 22

mitral valve in, 89
myocardial infarction and, 107
myxomas and, 97
nicotine addiction and, 18
nuclear stress tests and, 191
obesity in, 32, 33
PCIs and, 170–171
peripartum cardiomyopathy
    and, 87–88
physician bias, CAD, and
    referral patterns for, 193–194
physician gender and cardiac
    catheterization for, 195–197
polycystic ovary syndrome and, 31
population of, in U.S., 231
predictive value of tests and, 120
Primary Pulmonary
    Hypertension and, 100
PTCA success rates and, 169
race, obesity and, 35
risk factors for heart disease
    specific to, 15
sedentary lifestyle and
    cardiovascular disease in, 38
smoking and, 16, 17
statins and, 156
stenting and mortality rate for, 170
Takotsubo cardiomyopathy
    and, 88
torsade de points and, 164
waist/hip ratio in, 34

Women physicians
    in Rome, 210
    at Salerno medical school, 214
Women's Health Initiative, 70
    Hormone study, 73
    Observational Study, 15
Women's Health Study, 44, 45
Women's Heart Foundation, web site
    for, 228
Women's Heart Study, of aspirin, 149
Women's movement, impact of, in
    medicine, 190
Wrinkling, premature, smoking and,
    18

X

Xanthoma, 23
X-ray view of heart, *4*

Z

Zebeta, 143
Zestril, 142
Zetia, 161
Zipes, Douglas, 185
Zocor, 153, 157
Zyban, 20